Acclaim for Charles Barber's

Comfortably Numb

"Unlike many other books that excoriate psychiatrists, pharmaceutical companies, and other portions of the medical establishment for giving primacy to medication over humaneness, Barber's *Comfortably Numb* is filled with time-tested solutions."

—*The Hartford Courant*

"Fascinating." —*Philadelphia Weekly*

"Barber's message is one of hard truth and hope."

—*Austin American-Statesman*

"Thoughtful and surprisingly entertaining."

—*Playboy*

"Engaging. . . . An excellent, readable book."

—PsychCentral

"A fine, informed writer on cultural history as well as neuroscience, psychotherapy, and economics, Barber convincingly argues against the overprescription of psychiatric drugs in the United States and sums up the history of U.S. psychiatry from the asylum to the community to glitzy but still elementary neuroscience. A blockbuster."

—*Library Journal* (starred review)

"A handy compendium of evidence for the belief that we are overmedicated. . . . The issue that Barber addresses, distinguishing the treatment of disease from what I have called 'cosmetic psychopharmacology,' remains important." —Peter D. Kramer, *Slate*

"*Comfortably Numb* chronicles the extraordinary psychopharmaceuticalization of everyday life that has arisen in recent years and appears to be growing apace. Charles Barber marks out the inconvenient truths on our path to emotional climate change but also offers alternatives to readers who wish to avoid pharmageddon."

—David Healy, author of *Let Them Eat Prozac*

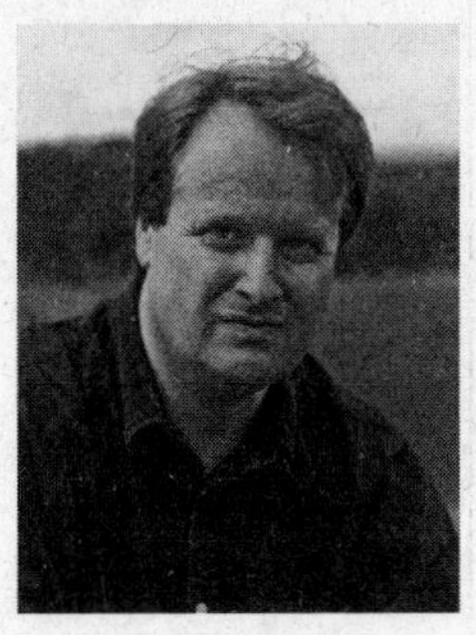

CHARLES BARBER

Comfortably Numb

Charles Barber was educated at Harvard and Columbia and worked for ten years in New York City shelters for the homeless mentally ill. The title essay in his first book, *Songs from the Black Chair*, won a 2006 Pushcart Prize, and his work has appeared in *The New York Times*, *The Washington Post*, and *Scientific American Mind*. He has been a guest on NPR's *Fresh Air* and *The Early Show* and is currently a lecturer in psychiatry at the Yale University School of Medicine and a senior executive with The Connection, a human and community development agency. He lives in Connecticut with his family.

www.charlesbarberwriting.com

Also by Charles Barber

Songs from the Black Chair: A Memoir of Mental Interiors

Comfortably Numb

Comfortably Numb

How Psychiatry Is Medicating a Nation

CHARLES BARBER

VINTAGE BOOKS
A Division of Random House, Inc.
New York

Fitchburg Public Library
5530 Lacy Road
Fitchburg, WI 53711

FIRST VINTAGE BOOKS EDITION, FEBRUARY 2009

Copyright © 2008 by Charles Barber

All rights reserved. Published in the United States by Vintage Books, a division of Random House, Inc., New York, and in Canada by Random House of Canada Limited, Toronto. Originally published in hardcover in the United States by Pantheon Books, a division of Random House, Inc., New York, in 2008.

Vintage and colophon are registered trademarks of Random House, Inc.

Grateful acknowledgment is made to the following for permission to reprint previously published material:

Random House, Inc.: Excerpt from "The Tenth Elegy" from *The Selected Poetry of Rainer Maria Rilke*, translated by Stephen Mitchell, copyright © 1982 by Stephen Mitchell. Reprinted by permission of Random House, Inc.

Guilford Publications, Inc.: Adapted version of the chart, "The Cognitive Model," from *Cognitive Therapy: Basics and Beyond* by Judith S. Beck, copyright © 1995 by Judith S. Beck; adapted version of the chart, "The Stages of Change Model," from *Addiction and Change: How Addictions Develop and Addicted People Recover* by Carlo C. DiClemente, Howard T. Blane, and Thomas R. Kosten, copyright © 2003 by Carlo C. DiClemente, Howard T. Blane, and Thomas R. Kosten. Reprinted by permission of Guilford Publications, Inc.

BMJ Publishing Group: Excerpt from "Scientists Find New Disease: Motivational Deficiency Disorder" by Ray Moynihan (*British Medical Journal*, April 1, 2006, vol. 332, page 745). Reprinted by permission of BMJ Publishing Group Limited.

The Library of Congress has cataloged the Pantheon edition as follows:
Barber, Charles.
Comfortably numb / how psychiatry is medicating a nation / Charles Barber.
p. cm.
Includes bibliographical references and index.
1. Mental illness—Chemotherapy—United States—History. 2. Psychotropic drugs—Marketing—United States—History. 3. Psychotropic drugs industry—Moral and ethical aspects—United States. 4. Biological psychiatry—United States—History. 5. Psychiatry—United States—History. 6. Deceptive advertising—United States. [DNLM: 1. Mental Disorders—Drug therapy—United States. 2. Drug Industry—United States. 3. Drug Therapy—Utilization—United States. 4. Psychiatry—Trends—United States. WM 402 B234c 2008] I. Title.
RC483.B28 2008
616.89'18—dc22 2007028541

Vintage ISBN: 978-0-307-27495-3

Author photograph © Amy Pierce
Book design by Soonyoung Kwon

www.vintagebooks.com

Printed in the United States of America
10 9 8 7 6 5 4 3 2

For Robert Coles, writer and teacher, and

for William J. Barber, scholar and father

A great part of both the strength and weakness of our national existence lies in the fact that Americans do not abide very quietly the evils of life. We are forever restlessly pitting ourselves against them, demanding changes, improvements, remedies, but not often with sufficient sense of the limits that the human condition will in the end insistently impose on us.

—RICHARD HOFSTADTER, *The Age of Reform*, 1955

There is always a well-known solution to every human problem—neat, plausible, and wrong.

—H. L. MENCKEN, *Prejudices: Second Series*, 1920

Contents

Foreword: "So Hip, So Quickly" xi

PART ONE
Neurons, Incorporated

ONE Who Medicated Iowa? 3
TWO The Commerce of Mood 22
THREE The Triumph of Biological Psychiatry 60
FOUR American Misery 100

PART TWO
A Series of Alternative Approaches

FIVE *Cogito, Ergo Sum* 139
SIX The Human Factor 168
SEVEN The Sea Snail Syndrome 191

Postscript: Emotional Rescue 211

Acknowledgments 227
Notes 231
Index 267

Foreword

"So Hip, So Quickly"

In 1988, almost by accident, I began working with homeless people suffering from mental illness in New York City. This was meant to be a short-term vocation, a year at most. But for the next fourteen years, I worked with the homeless mentally ill in Manhattan in a variety of settings—first on the streets, then in shelters, then in supportive residential programs. All of my clients suffered from, as the psychiatric textbooks put it, "severe and persistent mental illness." That is, they were diagnosed with various forms of schizophrenia, extreme mood complications such as bipolar disorder and major depression, and a range of personality disorders. Most of my clients had been or were addicted to some combination or other of alcohol, heroin, crack, cocaine, benzodiazepines, and PCP. A very large percentage had chronic physical ailments like diabetes, HIV, and hepatitis. Despite the rather remarkable burden of their collective afflictions, my clients were also often engaging, interesting, and without exception astonishingly resilient.

To quell their unruly moods and their troublesome delusions and hallucinations, my patients were taking all manner of psychiatric medications. Some of these medications had been around since the 1950s and 1960s—mood stabilizers like lithium, antipsychotics such as Haldol and Thorazine—while others, at the time, were brand-new, with strange and exotic names like Prozac, Paxil, and Zoloft. Each year over the course of the 1990s, new psychiatric medications were introduced and consumed en masse by my clients. Some of these new medications arrived with great fanfare and extremely high expectations. In particular, a class of agents called "atypical antipsychotics"—Risperdal, Clozaril, and Zyprexa are the best known—had been shown in early clinical studies to be far superior to the Haldols and the Thorazines. Overnight, it seemed, almost all patients were converted to these new drugs, as well as new-generation antidepressants and mood stabilizers. It was not at all unusual for my clients to be taking three, four, five, or six different types of psychiatric drugs in a given day—a combination not unlike the number of street drugs many of them had once been addicted to.

I am not a psychiatrist. My job was first as a counselor at, and then director of, a number of clinical and residential programs, and finally as a senior administrator at social services agencies and a researcher at medical schools. But I became oddly enthralled by the ongoing parade of medications that entered my clients' mouths (and sometimes their arms, via injection). I became deeply immersed in the sheer zeitgeist of all that was involved in their ever more complex pharmacological regimens: from the monthly filling of their multiple prescriptions (which would have cost hundreds and hundreds of dollars if not paid for by Medicaid); to the cheerful colors and happy-sounding, near-poetic names of the drugs (and the colors become more vibrant and the names more poetic as the 1990s wore on); to the regular visits of perky drug reps ready to hand out free meals, pens, calendars, and coffee cups to anybody who would listen; and, not least, to the complicated and broadly variable impact of the drugs on my clients' symptoms, personalities, and physical health. The influence of the drugs ranged greatly: from near-miraculous apparent "cures"; to therapeutic numbing, to no effects whatsoever; to, in one case, a near-fatal attack.

In the late 1980s, when I told people outside the field about my work—say, friends at cocktail parties in suburban, upper-middle-class Connecticut, where I grew up—no one seemed to quite comprehend what I did for a living. The prevailing tenor of these conversations was one of confusion. It would require real effort on my part to explain to these highly educated, eminently bourgeois people the nature of the problems which my clients faced. Sipping white wine, my friends and the friends of my parents struggled to grasp terms like *bipolar disorder* and *schizophrenia*. If I happened to mention the medications my clients were taking, the names fell upon barely comprehending ears. (Or I would be asked, in so many words: "Those are those zombie meds that they gave out in the old mental hospitals, aren't they?") It was also evident that these professors and lawyers and businesspeople, while not lacking in compassion, suspected my clients of having taken way too many drugs and/or being possessed of a seedy moral shiftlessness. The consensus was that while my clients were no doubt victims of multiple forms of injustice, their own characterological defects or weakness was the primary cause of their problems. I was sure that I was suspected of slumming—of immersing myself in a noble but deeply unsuitable venture for someone of my background and education. Returning to my work on the streets and in the shelters of New York City, I felt that what I was doing was at the very margins of American society.

But by the end of the 1990s, at these same cocktail parties, not only did people enthusiastically appreciate what I did, they were likely to share with me in no longer hushed tones that their friend or son or "someone very close to me" was suffering from depression or some other major psychiatric illness, and many were taking a number of the same drugs my clients were. Words like *Prozac* and *Paxil* and *lithium* were tossed around along with the salted peanuts and the shrimp. Upon learning the nature of my work, people would gather around, and I would be solicited for advice on various technical questions, like how long it took for Zoloft to fully enter the bloodstream and the advantages of Depakote as compared to lithium, or whether a neighbor's behavior was classically bipolar or merely hypomanic. Everyone seemed to be filled with a new and abrupt compassion for my clients, who, it was now universally agreed, were—of course! how could it be otherwise!—suffering from chemical imbalances and inner torments that, while unseen, were as physiological and real as diabetes or cancer. My career choice was to be applauded, and it was universally agreed that I was engaged in something important and meaningful. Even the terminology had changed: I no longer worked in shelters with psychotic people but in the brand-new shiny field of "Mental Health."

There was of course nothing unique about the cocktail parties I was attending. These same discussions and attitudinal changes were flowing vigorously through the popular culture. During the 1990s, mental illness became highly visible and quite suddenly almost chic. One celebrity after another confessed to their long-secret psychiatric anguishes. A movie about a genius with paranoid schizophrenia, *A Beautiful Mind*, won multiple Oscars. Radio talk show hosts began to talk semiknowledgeably about borderline personality disorder and the differences between SSRI and MAOI antidepressants. The wife of the vice president of the United States, Tipper Gore, revealed in a national op-ed that she had suffered from clinical depression.[1] In 1999, Bill Clinton convened a high-profile summit meeting on the nation's mental health, and his surgeon general released the first report on that topic. Even George W. Bush, not typically known for his progressive stances, issued his own remarkably forward-looking report on mental health in 2002 and publicly supported "mental health parity"—equality in the insurance coverage of physical and mental ailments. Bush declared: "Political leaders, health-care professionals, and all Americans must understand and send this message: mental disability is not a scandal—it is an illness."[2] In a reflection of how much support for "mental health" has moved to the fore, in 2004 California passed Proposition 63, "the millionaires for mental health tax," by which citizens with personal income over $1 million were levied an additional tax to fund the expansion of public psychiatric services. Over the course of the 1990s and into the 2000s, there was widespread optimism about the new medications and about the curative possibilities of advances in psychiatry in general. I would attend psychiatric conferences and hear breathless predictions that the genetic causes of schizophrenia would be identified within a decade, and a cure would follow not long thereafter.

But the biggest sign of the newfound acceptance of and fascination with the new biological psychiatry lay within our own bloodstreams. Each year more and more Americans were taking psychiatric medications, particularly the SSRI (selective serotonin reuptake inhibitor) antidepressants like Zoloft, Paxil, and Prozac.

What started as a drip developed into a stream, a river, and then a torrent. Introduced to the market in 1988, Prozac appeared on the cover of *Newsweek* in 1990 ("A Breakthrough Drug for Depression"); was the subject of a best-selling and extremely influential book, Peter Kramer's *Listening to Prozac* in 1993; graced, again, in 1994 the *Newsweek* cover, this time with even greater claims ("Shy? Forgetful? Anxious? Fearful? Obsessed? How Science Will Let You Change Your Personality with a Pill"); and exceeded a billion dollars in sales in 1995.[3] Prozac famously launched the concept of "cosmetic psychopharmacology," or the use of drugs for people who are patently not ill. In an oft-quoted passage from *Listening to Prozac*, Peter Kramer wrote, "With Prozac I had seen patient after patient become . . . better than well. Prozac seemed to give social confidence to the habitually timid, to make the sensitive brash, to lend the introvert the social skills of a salesman." In addressing lifestyle issues rather than actual diseases, Prozac vastly expanded its market base and paved the way for a succession of lifestyle-enhancing medications—Viagra, most notably; Lipitor and other cholesterol medications; a series of other psychiatric drugs—which have overwhelmingly driven Big Pharma's profits over the last decade.

It worked beyond anybody's expectations. Sales of Prozac hit $2 billion in 1998.[4] In 2002, more than 11 percent of American women and 5 percent of American men were taking antidepressants, which amounts to about 25 million people.[5] After its introduction, Prozac became the best-selling drug in the history of the pharmaceutical industry up until that point.[6] No one knows how many people in America have tried antidepressants at one point or another, but given that only about a quarter of people who start a course of antidepressants continue to take them for longer than ninety days,[7] it is entirely conceivable that 60, 70, 80 million Americans may have taken them.

And despite an FDA warning in 2004 of the increased risk of suicidal behavior for young people associated with SSRI antidepressants and a great deal of public-relations bloodying of Big Pharma in 2006 and 2007, antidepressant use actually went up during that period. In 2006, 227 million antidepressant prescriptions were dispensed to Americans—more than any other class of medication—and up by *30 million* prescriptions since 2002.[8]

While there were many positive aspects to this shift (the most important being the reduction in stigma toward the people with whom I worked), the rapidity with which the transformation occurred and the certainty with which the new consensus was endorsed were slightly bizarre to me. While the new attitudes about psychiatry were a vast improvement, representing a far more enlightened and realistic set of beliefs about what mental illness is really like, they also seemed in some ways just as sketchily and prematurely arrived at as the earlier convictions. There was, in short, a newfound *faddishness* about the whole phenomenon. It felt as if, overnight, the divide between my homeless, mentally ill clients and the wealthy, prosperous denizens of suburban America—who had heretofore lived in such separate worlds that it was hard for me to fathom that they occupied the same continent—was gone. The cocktail party set and the homeless mentally ill were now inextricably linked, not least by the pharmaceuticals that ran through their bloodstreams.

Many of the greatest advances in psychiatry in the last two decades have actually occurred outside the realm of psychotropic medications: in particular, a series of elegant and subtle refinements in social and therapeutic techniques, such as cognitive-behavioral therapy (CBT), that have produced outcomes that would be the envy of many if not most drug trials. For example, CBT has been shown to be as effective or possibly more effective than antidepressants in treating mild and moderate depression, and with a significantly lower recurrence rate.[9] CBT has also been used with a high degree of effectiveness for a dizzying number of conditions—among them, bulimia, hypochondriasis, obsessive-compulsive disorder, substance abuse, posttraumatic stress disorder, even as a proven means of reducing criminal behavior. Cognitive-behavioral treatments have been shown in analyses to reduce criminal recidivism by 25 percent.[10] One can only imagine the hype that would surround a pill if it was found to reduce criminal behavior at such a rate. Ads for "Pacify," as it might be called, would dominate the airwaves, and the public debate, for years.

Furthermore, two innovative treatment approaches—the Stages of Change model and Motivational Interviewing—have provided an entirely new paradigm of how caregivers conceive of the process by which people change and how to motivate them to do so. Their tenets, in a nutshell, are that change should be viewed as a cyclical process rather than a linear one; the job of changing is the responsibility of the patient, not the caregiver, thereby putting the recipient of care "in charge" and reversing the centuries-old hierarchical construct of the doctor-patient relationship; and the approach that the caregiver takes in assisting the client to change must vary according to the client's "stage of change"—that is, their insight and motivation to move forward on a particular problem. The positive outcomes of these various approaches in alleviating some of the most intractable of human problems—such as addictions and the most severe mental illnesses, like schizophrenia—have been proven repeatedly. But no one outside the field even knows about these alternative approaches. Why should they? There are no products associated with these developments to sell to the masses, no billions to be made on Wall Street.

Furthermore, research on the brain has revealed the unexpected "plasticity" of the organ—i.e., its capacity to change its function and structure throughout life. Brain imaging has shown that social and psychological experiences exert measurable changes in the brain. Specifically, learning and social experience—such as psychotherapy, for what is psychotherapy other than a particularly intensive form of learning?—are capable of producing changes in the brain at the level of neuronal and synaptic connections. There is no longer any doubt that psychotherapy can change the brain at functional and structural levels. That is, in perhaps the greatest irony of the neuro revolution, psychotherapy can be viewed as a "biological" treatment, along with pharmaceutical approaches.

But these exciting, if at times complex and nuanced, advances have gone almost completely unnoticed by the media and the public, and underappreciated even within the field of psychiatry. In the last two decades, there has been a tremendous bias in academic psychiatry against psychological and social forms of inquiry. The psychosocial realm is tolerated but often barely so—viewed as well-intentioned and sort of cute, but ultimately and soundly relegated to the margins, literally and figuratively. The programs at which I have worked at the Yale and Columbia medical schools that were engaged in such social approaches were typically way off-campus, sometimes near derelict settings.

In this era, one could hardly get an article published in an academic journal of psychiatry that was purely qualitative (i.e., didn't include statistics), or that told the story of an individual patient, or that included any personal thoughts or feelings on the part of the authors about the people or the work they were engaged with. All that would be deemed not appropriately robust for the new standards of the profession. In our particularly American zeal for simple explanations, quick fixes, and overwhelming the enemy with technology, we've too quickly lost sight of the centrality of social and environmental factors. And despite undeniable progress in the pharmacological realm, the enduring truth is that the human factor, and the human approach, remains critical to healing.

Meanwhile, back in the shelters in New York City, my clients remained essentially unchanged by the pharmacological advances which had surrounded them during the 1990s. In the early 2000s, they were suffering from the same exact set of monstrous afflictions that had beset them a decade earlier. The new medications had brought some relief, and in a few cases dramatic improvements, but in general they were a disappointment. Analyses over the last couple of years have shown that the new medications are no more effective, or only minimally more effective, than the old ones, while often costing at least ten times as much. Additionally, some of the new antipsychotics cause rapid and intense weight gain, leading to high rates of diabetes. Two massive government studies released in 2006 on the real-world efficacy (as opposed to that reported in clinical trials) of both antidepressants and antipsychotics showed that most patients do not get better taking the drugs. Only about a third of patients taking antidepressants, for example, improved dramatically after a first trial.[11] For antipsychotics, the story was even worse. Three-quarters of study participants stopped taking their medication before the end of eighteen months.[12] Said Robert Freedman, M.D., editor in chief of the *American Journal of Psychiatry:* "The results of STAR*D [the depression trial] continue to be sobering. By the third wave of the study, the rate of remission continues to be quite low, which underscores the persistence of depression, and its resistance to current treatments."[13]

In some ways, things were actually worse by 2000. The emergence of managed care—the handmaiden of the medication revolution—had severely shortened hospital stays. Under managed care, psychiatric hospitalization came to be viewed not as an opportunity to work on treatment issues or to arrive at a thoughtful discharge plan, but primarily as a place to tinker with medications. Once a medication regimen was arrived at, and patients were no longer considered unsafe, they were out, sometimes on the streets. My clients were routinely hospitalized and rehospitalized, and discharged and redischarged, always before they were ready. This caused incalculable confusion and pain.

No, it was the people at the cocktail parties who had changed—not my clients.

Going back to New York, I would wonder: *How did this happen, and in such a short time? How did attitudes about mental illness—no, "mental health"—change so quickly?*

Back in the shelters, I would wonder: *How did biological psychiatry get to be so omnipresent, so powerful, so hip, so quickly?*

PART ONE

Neurons, Incorporated

CHAPTER ONE

Who Medicated Iowa?

By all accounts, Winterset, Iowa—population about five thousand, located in the southern and central part of the state—is a wonderful place to live. The local newspaper regularly features such items as:

> Justin Decker spent Friday night with his great-grandparents, Ralph and Georgena Breakenridge.
>
> Cindy Porter, Rachel Miller and Angela Holtry attended a birthday party for Jean Wagner on Saturday night at the VFW hall in Winterset.[1]

The town's Web site proclaims:

> It's a great place to be! . . . If you live around the corner, or halfway around the world, we invite you to visit and take a closer look at what our GREAT town has to offer. We have excellent reasons to refer to Winterset as a GREAT place to to

> [*sic*] live and raise a family. Those fortunate enough to call our town "Home" tell about the benefits of living in a place where quality of life and economic prosperity go hand in hand.[2] . . . We hope you'll visit and see what we mean when we say we live in a GREAT place."

Winterset, also known as the "City of Parks," is located at the junction of Routes 169 and 92, close (but not too close for the tranquility of its residents) to Interstate 80, which traverses the state. The main thoroughfares in Winterset are West Summit Street and John Wayne Drive. Wayne was born here—as Marion Robert Morrison—in a modest house in 1907. Other streets are named after presidents: Fillmore, Buchanan, Jefferson, Washington. There are sixteen churches in town: denominations include Methodist, Evangelical, Lutheran, the Disciples of Christ, Catholic, Presbyterian, Gospel, Baptist, Jehovah's Witness, Presbyterian, as well as the Manjushri Tibetan Center. You can buy used cars at Merrill's Garage; books at the Corner Bookstore; and Iowa Amish baskets and jams at the Screen Door General Store. The celebrated quilters Marianne Fons and Liz Porter run a quilting supply store at 54 Court Avenue, on the south side of Winterset's historic town square. Marianne and Liz host "America's #1 quilting show" *Fons & Porter's Love of Quilting* on public television. They are also owners and editors of *Love of Quilting* magazine, which has a circulation of about 300,000. The Red Delicious apple was originally cultivated by a farmer near Winterset in 1880, and to celebrate that fact, the region holds an annual Apple Days festival every Autumn.

This is breadbasket America. Madison County, of which Winterset is the county seat, has almost one thousand farms. There are 61,000 acres of corn and 63,000 acres of soybeans. In a typical year, 110,000 hogs and 23,000 head of cattle are sold in the county.[3] The area is famous for its covered bridges. The novel and film *The Bridges of Madison County* was set in and filmed in and around Winterset.

Between May 25 and 27, 2007, Winterset celebrated the one hundredth birthday of John Wayne. The festivities included the groundbreaking of the John Wayne Birthplace Museum with Wayne's son Ethan in attendance; the John Wayne Birthday Wild West Revue, complete with a live stagecoach robbery, with appearances by Buffalo Bill and Annie Oakley. There was an old-fashioned hometown parade and cowboy symposia with Wayne's co-stars Dean Smith, Gregg Palmer, and Edward Faulkner, and a performance by a cowboy band, Riders in the Sky.

If anybody appreciated the virtues of Winterset, it was Ronald Reagan. The Gipper passed through on the campaign trail in 1984, proclaiming "It's great to be back in Iowa, and it's great to be here in Madison County and in Winterset, the birthplace of a man who was a great patriot and a close friend, John Wayne. When I think of the Duke and all the other great Americans who've claimed this state as their home, I have to agree with the writer who said, 'Iowa is top-choice America, America cut thick and prime.' "[4]

But apparently all is not entirely well in Winterset. There are various signs of trouble and unease. On September 3, 2002, one of the famous covered bridges, the Cedar Bridge, was destroyed by fire. The sheriff's department suspects arson and continues to offer a $41,000 award for information that leads to the arrest and conviction of the perpetrator. In 2006, the Winterset Git-N-Go convenience store was robbed of an undetermined amount of money by an unidentified white middle-aged male. And in March 2007, for two weeks in a row no one bothered to show up at the public hearings to review the town's $11 million 2007–2008 budget.[5]

Wellmark Blue Cross and Blue Shield (which has the interesting and perhaps ironic slogan "You Just Can't Beat the Blues™), the state's largest insurance company, reports on its Web site that in 2002, *16 percent* of the citizens of Winterset were taking antidepressants. Apparently, one in six of these bankers, farmers, mechanics, quilters, and housewives, and of these Buddhist, Presbyterians, and Baptists of Winterset are feeling so miserable that they feel they need help. What is compelling one in six of these generally prosperous and stable citizens to go to their doctor, get a prescription, and go to the Montross

Pharmacy on North First Avenue to find something to make them feel better?

And Winterset is by no means alone. Other towns in Iowa have similar usage rates (or utilization, as they like to say in managed care) of antidepressants: for Ames it is 17.5 percent; for Grinnell, 16 percent; Des Moines, 16 percent; Cedar Rapids, 16 percent; Anamosa, Red Oak, and Perry, 15 percent. The national average for Blue Cross and Blue Shield subscribers in 2000, by the way, was a still rather shocking 10.7 percent.[6]

It has been widely observed that the SSRIs put many people at a sort of remove from reality, a distance from the self. I've seen SSRIs block out both the good and the bad, numbing us to the pandemonium of life. I have noticed that people who take the drugs to attempt to redress ordinary life problems, rather than serious depression, are more prone to this sanitizing flatness. The emotional highs and lows are excised from experience, and one exists in a slightly foggy middle ground. Some people said that they have a sense of observing themselves going through their day, going through the motions, seeing themselves from afar. They feel flat, at times unresponsive. They function; they don't get too excited or too upset. They get by. They come to inhabit an inauthentic and less challenging existence and embrace a uniquely American form of emotional sanitation. Or as one veteran of Paxil observed: "I hate this feeling . . . this feeling of not being able to feel."[7] When going off the drugs, many people say they are happy to feel the highs and the lows again.

One wonders: What is going on in the heart of America—in America "thick and prime"? What miseries are residing within the chamber of the human heart in Winterset?

Why did Winterset want to get numb?

The people of the town may not know it, but Winterset is just one outpost, if a particularly prolific and lucrative one, of an economic and cultural phenomenon that has been building steadily since the 1988 arrival of Prozac, followed later by its cousins Zoloft and Paxil. The one in six people of Winterset who take SSRIs and other antidepressants represent just one minuscule piece—one nail perhaps, or a little screw—of a towering, looming structure that has been building and growing and enlarging inexorably and relentlessly over the course of the 1990s. The construction of "the Empire of Serotonin," as I like to call it, was a masterpiece of marketing, as well as a formidable testament to the ease and rapidity with which massive sociological change can occasionally be realized.

The only comparable product in recent American history, in terms of influence on both the market and the popular mindset, has been the sports utility vehicle. In fact the SUV story and SSRI story have remarkable similarities: both grew into iconic products of their age, and both represent in their respective industries the most extraordinary kind of overkill, or what marketers call "overperformance," the gap, or disconnect, between a product's maximal capabilities and what is needed for everyday, real-world use.[8] SUVs may well be able to pull three tons up the Himalayas, but most people need them only to get to Wal-Mart at three in the afternoon. Similarly, antidepressants can be truly life-saving for people with severe and disabling mental illness, but when ingested by people attempting to manage the daily problems of living or garden-variety existential angst, let alone "social anxiety disorder" (what most people would call shyness) and separation anxiety in dogs (both FDA-approved uses of SSRIs), their efficacy and their risk-reward calculus become rapidly more dubious. In this regard, SSRIs and SUVs, along with other distinctly American technologies like cell phones and fast food, are all the same: useful when you really need them but mainly unnecessary and vastly and indiscriminately over-used.

The very existence of the Serotonin Empire was quite remarkable, given that before the antidepressants arrived, depression was considered a rare disease, affecting about 1 percent of the population (as opposed to 10 to 15 percent of the population today); that after early clinical trials, Prozac was nearly shelved by Eli Lilly and almost never saw the light of day; and that, early on, German regulators concluded about the drug: "Considering the benefit and the risk, we think this preparation totally unsuitable for the treatment of depression."[9] Prozac was actually killed in development seven times before Lilly ultimately allowed it to go to market.[10] When David Wong, Prozac's codiscoverer, wrote an article on Prozac, before its entry on the market, intended for the journal *Science*, it was rejected by an editor who said there was no general interest in the topic.[11] But the residents of Winterset, looking at themselves in the mirror of their bathroom vanities at 10 p.m. on a Tuesday, and swallowing their Prozac or Paxil or Zoloft, were happily oblivious of this. Caught up in the national fervor of what the anthropologist T. M. Luhrmann has politely described as "psychopharmacological overenthusiasm," the residents stood in line at the Montross Pharmacy and swallowed their pills at night.[12]

The size and reach of the psychiatric drug industry is staggering. It is far, far greater than most psychiatric practitioners realize and certainly greater than the drug companies would want you to know. There are various ways to measure the dimensions of the enterprise:

- 33 million Americans were prescribed at least one psychiatric drug in 2004, up from 21 million in 1997.[13]
- The spending on antidepressants rose from $5.1 billion in 1997 to $13.5 billion in 2006; and on antipsychotics from $1.3 billion in 1997 to 11.5 billion in 2006.[14]
- The third-best-selling antidepressant, Lexapro, has been on the market only since 2002. But 15 million Americans have already taken it.[15]
- Nine percent of American teens have been prescribed drugs for depression.[16]
- The products are not limited to adults, and not even to humans. In 2002, 11 million antidepressant prescriptions were written for American children and adolescents.[17] Before 1990, outside of the occasional use of Ritalin, the medicating of kids was just about taboo. Clomicalm (known as Anafranil when taken by humans) is approved by the FDA for separation anxiety for dogs. To increase their appeal for these segments of the market, Prozac and Paxil come in mint- and orange-flavored liquids, respectively, and Clomicalm is meat-

flavored. A Los Angeles veterinarian estimates that 5 percent of the cats and dogs in his practice are taking psychotropic agents for their behavior.[18]

- Zoloft's American sales—$3.1 billion in 2005—exceeded those of Tide detergent that same year.[19, 20]
- The worldwide sales of one drug for schizophrenia, Zyprexa—$4.7 billion in 2006—were greater than the revenue generated by the Levi Strauss Co.[21]

Accompanying the sales of the drugs (indeed what has made the sales and ingestion of the drugs possible, at least in part) has been an equally dramatic attitude shift toward mental dysfunction on the part of Americans. As the drugs have sailed to the top of the charts, mental illness and psychiatry have gone from being taboo subjects to becoming almost chic.

Tony Soprano takes Prozac, lithium, and Xanax (and his mother, Livia, took Prozac, and AJ, his son, is put on Lexapro, a newer antidepressant, in the show's last season.) Dr. Phil is a star. Eminem is on antidepressants. Lorraine Bracco (who happens to play Tony Soprano's psychiatrist) and Halle Berry suffer from depression; Brooke Shields, from postpartum depression; and David Beckham, from obsessive-compulsive disorder. Hardly a week goes by without a celebrity revealing—usually in some well-chosen commercial format—their long-secret psychiatric disorder. High-profile confessors of recent years include Jane Pauley, whose revelation of bipolar disorder in a book and TV special was timed with the launch of her daytime talk show, and three-time Grammy winner Shawn Colvin, whose tour was sponsored by GlaxoSmithKline, the makers of the folksinger's antidepressant of choice, Wellbutrin XL. The favored confessional platform is *The Oprah Winfrey Show*, where celebrities like Colvin and Linda Hamilton, the tough female action star of *The Terminator* movies, divulge their inner torments on shows called "Depressed, Mentally Ill, and Famous." Even sports figures have proclaimed their biochemical deficiencies: Ricky Williams, formerly the NFL's leading rusher, and Terry Bradshaw, four-time Super Bowl champion, paired up to do ads for Paxil. (Williams claims that Paxil cured his anxiety, and Bradshaw his depression.) Julie Krone, Hall of Fame jockey, has endorsed Zoloft. Picabo Street, gold medal skier, has written about her depression.

Prozac alone has inspired a theatrical play *(Prozac Sisters)* and a video game *(Virtual Prozac)*[22] and has supplied the opening premise of a novel, Matthew Sharpe's *The Sleeping Father.* (The father takes too many antidepressants and goes into a coma.) There is a new magazine, *bp* (underwritten by Pfizer and Bristol-Myers Squibb), offering hope for people suffering from bipolar disorder. *Monk*, a show about a detective with obsessive-compulsive disorder who uses his illness adaptively to perceive things that normal people can't, is one of the most popular programs on cable television and has received a gaggle of Screen Actors Guild, Emmy, and Edgar awards. Some of the more appealing films of recent vintage—*As Good as It Gets*, *Girl, Interrupted*, *Good Will Hunting*, and *Matchstick Men*—have offered thoughtful, generally realistic portrayals of mental illness through characters played by superstar actors Jack Nicholson, Angelina Jolie, Matt Damon, and Nicolas Cage. Leonardo DiCaprio, in playing Howard Hughes in Martin Scorsese's *The Aviator*, not only portrayed Hughes's obsessive-compulsive tendencies brilliantly, but in promoting the movie acknowledged having a form of OCD himself. DiCaprio and Scorsese further demonstrated their sympathy for the cause by previewing the movie at a neuropsychiatric institute. *The Aviator* is the most recent of just a handful of movies (the other shining example is *A Beautiful Mind*) in cinema history that portray mental illness in full-bodied, nuanced, and even heroic terms. DiCaprio's Hughes and Russell Crowe's John Nash struggle powerfully with and often overcome their crippling illnesses. They present characters that are charming, brilliant, and sexy, in addition to being seriously disturbed. Both movies were rewarded with a slew of Oscar nominations.

In recent years, in fact, one's chances of getting nominated for an Oscar are greatly enhanced by playing a character experiencing mental dysfunction. In almost every year over the last decade, actors have either been nominated for or won Oscars for portraying a psychiatric disorder. Here's the list of actors and the putative diagnoses of the characters they portrayed:

2006	Jackie Earle Haley	*Little Children*	pedophilia
2005	Felicity Huffman	*Transamerica*	gender identity disorder
2004	Leonardo DiCaprio	*The Aviator*	obsessive-compulsive disorder
2004	Charlize Theron	*Monster*	posttraumatic stress disorder
2003	Tim Robbins	*Mystic River*	posttraumatic stress disorder; major depressive disorder with psychotic features
2002	Nicole Kidman	*The Hours*	major depressive disorder
2001	Russell Crowe	*A Beautiful Mind*	schizophrenia, paranoid type
	Sean Penn	*I Am Sam*	pervasive developmental disorder (mental retardation)
	Judi Dench	*Iris*	Alzheimer's disease
2000	Ed Harris	*Pollock*	bipolar disorder
1999	Angelina Jolie	*Girl, Interrupted*	borderline personality disorder
1997	Matt Damon	*Good Will Hunting*	antisocial disorder
	Jack Nicholson	*As Good as It Gets*	obsessive-compulsive disorder
1996	Geoffrey Rush	*Shine*	schizophrenia
	Billy Bob Thornton	*Sling Blade*	pervasive developmental disorder
1995	Brad Pitt	*12 Monkeys*	schizophrenia
	Nicholas Cage	*Leaving Las Vegas*	major depressive disorder; alcohol dependence
1994	Tom Hanks	*Forrest Gump*	pervasive developmental disorder
	Nigel Hawthorne	*The Madness of King George*	psychotic disorder
1993	Leonardo DiCaprio	*What's Eating Gilbert Grape*	pervasive developmental disorder

There is no other period in Hollywood history in which mental instability has been so regularly—or so well—portrayed. The depiction of craziness or mental impairment used to make the occasional appearance in the Hollywood of the 1930s through the 1970s—*The Lost Weekend*, *The Three Faces of Eve*, *The Snake Pit*—but now, clearly, it is an annual affair. Every A-list actor, it seems, has to take their shot playing a mentally retarded or crazy person.

In addition, the nature of the portrayal has changed. Until the last decade, Hollywood offered two paradigms of mental instability: the kindly mentally impaired person, suffering from some vaguely defined but nonetheless manifestly organic neurological disease *(Rain Man*, *Awakenings)*, or the homicidal over-the-top psychotic *(Psycho*, *Taxi Driver)*. But the last decade has brought depictions, sometimes even accurate ones, of specific disorders—schizophrenia, bipolar disorder, and depression—and their treatments. Hollywood has, in other words, discovered diagnosis and nuance. *Shine*, *A Beautiful Mind*, *As Good as It Gets*, *Good Will Hunting*, and *Girl, Interrupted* have all presented characters that are ill but talented, impaired but not stupid, troubled but attractive. The drugs themselves have become protagonists in recent movies. The plots of *Garden State* and *Michael Clayton* (both hailed by critics as representative films of our times) are set in motion when their characters no longer have access to or choose to take their psychiatric medications.

Another reflection of the newly upscale image of mental illness is the distance between portrayals of madness by the same actor during different decades. Jack Nicholson, in the '70s, played an obsessive and psychotic writer who wants to murder his family *(The Shining)*; in the '90s, he played an obsessive writer who is well-medicated, productive, wealthy, charming (albeit eccentrically so), and able to bed a woman half his age *(As Good as It Gets)*. Robert De Niro, in playing Travis Bickle in *Taxi Driver* in the '70s, delivered perhaps the most viscerally terrifying portrayal of psychosis in film history; in the '90s, in *Analyze This*, he played a mob boss afflicted with anxiety and depression who seeks out psychiatric treatment, which is successful, allowing him to feel both less disturbed *and* maintain his virility as a Mafioso. Gone by the wayside, too, in the new era is the mass-murdering, out-of-control, floridly dangerous psychotic, or psycho, as Hitchcock defined it. Even the word *psycho* has a dated, '70s pre-diagnostic ring to it.

Even psychiatrists, a longtime media whipping boy, are now sometimes favorably portrayed. The prime-time dramas *E.R.*, *Judging Amy*, *Law and Order*, *The West Wing*, *House*, and *Grey's Anatomy* have featured psychiatrists and psychologists who are *not* idiots, a rarity in the history of movies and television. (It used to be said that the positive portrayals of psychiatrists showed them sleeping with their patients, while the negative portrayals had them both sleeping with and then killing their patients.) Some—by no means all—of the shrinks in these TV dramas are smart and attractive and stable; they often deliver essential testimony or clinical information that helps the patient or solves the crime.

In particular, the psychiatrist played by B. D. Wong on *Law and Order* is portrayed as a kind of sage in profiling and predicting the behavior of suspects. He has the distinction of being both smart and street-smart.

In the new millennium, there can be a steep price if one portrays mental illness too harshly. In 2000, ABC introduced *Wonderland*, a prime-time drama set in a big city psychiatric emergency room, thinly based on Bellevue. The first episode featured a man with schizophrenia wildly shooting six people in Times Square. After being brought to the ER, he stabbed a pregnant doctor. In the next episode, the patient committed suicide. Alarmed at this portrayal of mental illness, the National Alliance for the Mentally Ill, 220,000 members strong, organized an aggressive public campaign against the show. In response, major sponsors—the drug companies AstraZeneca and Novartis, as well as Johnson & Johnson, Scotts Company, and Staples—withdrew their support. *Wonderland* was gone after two episodes.[23]

The trend continued in 2007, when General Motors, Volkswagen, and Washington Mutual all ran TV commercials that depicted depressive feelings and suicidal behavior, albeit in satirical ways. In the GM ad, which appeared during the Super Bowl broadcast, an assembly-line robot hurls itself off a bridge after committing an error; in the Washington Mutual spot, despondent bankers are poised to jump off a building; and in the VW ad, a man is about to jump off a ledge until he learns that he can buy a new VW for under $17,000. Mental health advocacy groups and the American Foundation for Suicide Prevention found the material offensive and wrote public letters to the corporations. All three companies capitulated, either dropping the ads from the airwaves or excising the egregious material.[24]

A study of newspaper reporting on mental illness showed that negative portrayals were reduced by half between 1989 and 1999, even though negative stories continued to outnumber positive ones.[25] Images and descriptions of mental illness are now omnipresent in the American media. Almost a third of American prime-time TV shows portrayed mental illness—whereas only 4 percent of British programs did.[26] After neglecting to feature a cover story on psychiatry or mental health between 1956 and 1983, *Time* has had eight such stories since

1990—four of them since 2001. We now conceive of national catastrophes as having both a physical and mental component. That is, there is first the reportage of the physical event—9/11, Katrina, Iraq War—and then there is the ensuing psychiatric fallout. Hence, *Time* asks, a year after Katrina, "Is New Orleans Having a Mental Health Breakdown?"[27] And CNN reports in 2007 that nearly a third of veterans returning from Iraq and Afghanistan come home with psychiatric or psychosocial ills. (Posttraumatic stress disorder led the way, accounting for almost half of all diagnoses, followed by anxiety, adjustment disorders, depression, and substance abuse disorders.)[28] In the aftermath of each of those events, there has been extensive media coverage, discussion, and debate about the mental health of the victims.

The fascination with and curiosity about antidepressants and depression on the part of the American public remains profound and unabashed. Based on Internet searches, antidepressants are much on the mind of Americans. Remarkably, almost a quarter of American Internet users have searched for mental health topics like depression and anxiety. As a category, mental health issues are searched for more often than immunizations, dental health, Medicare or Medicaid, sexual health information, or problems with drugs and alcohol.[29] In July 2006, of the ten most popular online searches for pharmaceutical and medical products, six concerned psychiatric drugs or psychiatric disease. (They were, in order, Lexapro, Cymbalta, Zoloft, Wellbutrin [an antianxiety agent], Effexor, and the illness of depression itself.)[30] Among people who have visited a medication site, depression is by far the most researched medical condition, with 2.9 million unique visitors over a three-month period in 2006. The next most researched conditions? Bipolar disorder and insomnia.[31]

To further the ascent of Prozac et al. it has helped immensely that there has been a simultaneous barrage of media messages and images in the last decade informing the public that behavior is biologically dictated. There is a daily drumbeat emanating from the TV and the newspapers informing us that behavior is genetic, hardwired, strictly biological. Newspapers, which hardly reported health news thirty years ago, report study after study showing that behavior is biologically inherited and determined. Headlines scream "Man's Genes Made Him Kill, His Lawyers Claim," or ask "Are Your Genes to Blame?" or simply state, as *The New York Times* did, "Lack Direction? Evaluate Your Brain's C.E.O.": "You can be truly smart and still struggle in life if you lack the ability to plan, [and] organize time and space . . . More and more neuroscientists are saying such puzzling underachievers may suffer from neurological abnormalities." (Where was that article when Holden Caulfield or Bart Simpson needed it?) When *The New York Times* ran an article on "flaming"—the impulsive sending of an e-mail message that is provocative or rude (called "online disinhibition effect" in the psychological literature)—the explanation of this activity was neuroscientific. Flaming was attributed to "a design flaw inherent in the interface between the brain's social circuitry"—more specifically, as the *Times* put it, the neural chatter between the orbitofrontal cortex and emotional centers like the amygdala—"and the online world."[32] And when a man in a New York City subway station jumped onto the tracks to save a stranger, the *Times* speculated that the reason had to do not with a sense of altruism or duty, but the way his brain was wired: "If it wasn't the Navy training that compelled Wesley Autrey to save a complete stranger, it was his well-oiled anterior cingulate, or his 'mirror neurons.' "[33] (Mirror neurons fire in response to observing the actions of another person and are thought to be sensitive even to the perceived intentions of another person. Calling them "cells that read minds," the *Times* seems to think there is little they are not capable of: "Mirror neurons reveal how children learn, why people respond to certain types of sports, dance, music and art, why watching media violence may be harmful, and why many men like pornography."[34]

The delivery of this information is unprecedented and relentless. In 2006, there was a spate of best-selling and high-profile books—*The Female Brain*, *Moral Minds: How Nature Designed Our Universal Sense of Right and Wrong*, *Breaking the Spell: Religion as a Natural Phenomenon*—that sought to explain highly complex issues (such as the difference between the sexes, our moral sense, spirituality) in biological and neurobiological terms. In just *one* edition of the *Times*, four articles appeared, each of which offered genetic and neurological explanations for behavior that a decade or two ago likely would have been analyzed in social or cultural terms:

- "A Biological Dig for the Roots of Language." Biologists, using genetic models, are outstripping linguists, who use traditional cultural models to understand how language developed.
- "Women in Black, Clues on Origins of Depression." Researchers may have explained the higher rates of depression among women by finding that a gene associated with the illness is far more common in women than men.
- "At the Movies: Brains in Sync." Brain scans showed that the same brain regions flashed on and off simultaneously in subjects watching dramatic scenes of a Clint Eastwood movie.
- "In Sex, Brain Studies Show, 'La Difference' Still Holds." Men and women who were shown erotic photographs reported equal levels of arousal, but brain scans showed that different regions of their brains lit up.[35]

This incessant *physicalizing* of behavior—which allows for a broken mind to be seen in roughly the same terms as a broken leg—has softened the image of psychological disturbance in general, and mental illness in particular. In this context, madness has, at times, become alluring and inviting and, at the very least, enormously popular. Sylvia Plath was remarkably prescient when she noted in her journal, while contemplating writing *The Bell Jar*, that "there's an increasing market for mental-hospital stuff."[36]

To be sure, the most common portrayal of mental illness, both in the movies and in the headlines, is still the violent schizophrenic. But given its sordid history, the image of mental illness has quite improbably and suddenly become nearly chic. We have seen an emergence of "psychiatric chic," akin to the "heroin chic" of models and downtown artists. Numerous undergraduates have told me that it's rather cool to be depressed at college these days (and all that goes with it, including public discussions of what antidepressants you're taking), at least as long as you grow out of it well before graduation. A poll of Harvard undergraduates found that 80 percent said they had felt depressed in the last year, and almost half had felt so depressed that it had been difficult to function. Harvard's mental health services have been overrun in recent years. Eighteen hundred graduates and undergraduates visit the university mental health services every year, and an additional six hundred fifty undergraduates receive therapy from the Bureau of Study Counsel. The bureau—originally founded to help students adjust to college life—has become a nearly full-time mental health center with thirteen clinicians in order to meet demand. ("This blows my mind!" said former Harvard president Larry Summers, apparently of the old school when it comes to matters of mental health, in response to these numbers.)[37]

It is in fact standard fare to be taking some sort of psychiatric drug in college these days. Professors have told me, after they've done informal polling of their students, that a third to a half have taken psychiatric drugs. The chief of Mental Health Services at Harvard wrote about antidepressants and attention deficit drugs in *The New England Journal of Medicine:* "Increasing numbers of students, and sometimes their families, request medication to provide an 'edge,' even if the students have no clinically significant impairment of functioning. They think of such drugs as safe 'brain steroids' that help to maximize performance with minimal risk, and they know the symptoms to describe in order to persuade a doctor to write a prescription."[38] A new science of retrospective diagnosis has emerged, whereby great historical figures such as Winston Churchill and Abraham Lincoln are diagnosed with particular mental illnesses decades and centuries after their deaths, and what's more, their infirmities are judged to be part of their greatness. *Lincoln's Melancholy: How Depression Challenged a President and Fueled His Greatness* is a recent best seller, leading to a *Time* cover story.[39] Another recent book, *The Hypomanic Edge: The Link Between Craziness and Success in America*, diagnosed Christopher Columbus, Alexander Hamilton,

Andrew Carnegie, Henry Ford, David O. Selznick, and the contemporary figures Ted Turner and Craig Venter with hypomania or bipolar disorder, and further postulated that if it were not for the excessive, even manic energy of these brilliant innovators of American capitalism, America wouldn't be the great country that it is today.

As a fellow mob boss says to Tony Soprano, assuring him that it's acceptable to be in therapy and to take Prozac: "There's no stigmata [*sic*] anymore." "I was seeing a therapist myself about a year ago," Paulie Walnuts tells Tony in one episode. "I had some issues."[40] In a somewhat related phenomenon, the use of the word *issues* as a substitute . . . no, a euphemism . . . for the word *problems* has entered universal usage. As in: we don't have problems anymore; we have "issues." So-and-so is not troubled; she has "issues." It's not that we don't get along with someone; we have "issues" with that person. It's another form of reduced "stigmata," yet another manifestation of political correctness applied to daily conflicts and dilemmas.

Cumulatively, the messages have hit their mark. Mental illness is not what it used to be in the eyes of the American public. In a poll done before the 2000 presidential election, voters didn't particularly care whether or not candidates had received psychiatric treatment or were taking antidepressants. Those issues—which proved explosive in 1972, when Democratic vice presidential candidate Thomas Eagleton withdrew from the race after it was revealed that he had undergone electroshock therapy for depression—hold little current interest for the public. There is a neat party distinction, by the way, when politicians get into psychic trouble: Democratic politicians and their wives tend to suffer from mental illness (Eagleton, Kitty Dukakis, Tipper Gore), and Republicans from drug abuse (Betty Ford, George W. Bush). Only one in five voters said the press should report that a presidential candidate is taking antidepressants, placing it below spouse abuse, income tax evasion, exaggerated military or academic record, ongoing or past affair, homosexuality, cocaine and marijuana use, or a past drinking problem as an area of concern.[41] In 2004, in a Rice University study of attitudes toward mental illness in the Houston area, respondents were twelve times more likely to ascribe the cause of mental illness to a brain disorder than to a character flaw.[42] In 1996, 38 percent of Americans viewed depression as a health problem, as opposed to a sign of personal weakness. By 2006, 72 percent saw depression as a health problem."[43] In general, Americans feel much closer to mental dysfunction. In 1957, one in five Americans reported having personal fears of an impending nervous breakdown; by 1996, it was one in four.

In this environment, then, it is not at all surprising that Americans think that they are much crazier than people in other countries. In 2004, the World Health Organization completed a study on the global prevalence of mental illness. Based on structured, in-home interviews, an extraordinary *26 percent* of Americans reported that they suffered from any type of psychiatric disorder in the prior year—far exceeding the rates of all of the other fifteen countries. By contrast, 5 percent of Nigerians, 8 percent of Italians, 9 percent of Germans, and 12 percent of Mexicans reported having a psychiatric disorder. (The only country that came close to the United States was perennially troubled Ukraine.) Americans described themselves as being particularly vulnerable to anxiety disorders and impulse-control disorders, reporting them at double the rates of every other country but Colombia and France. Almost 8 percent of Americans reported having suffered from a serious mental disorder, a rate about three times higher than any other developed country in the survey.[44] In reporting the story, *The New York Times* stated, bluntly, about Americans: "Most Will Be Mentally Ill at Some Point, Study Says."[45] "We lead the world in a lot of good things, but we're also leaders in this one particular domain that we'd rather not be," said the study's lead author.[46]

Americans have responded to what's in the air, and on the air, around them. They are deeply immersed in craziness. They take drugs for their perceived insanity at rates far exceeding any other country; they make movies and watch TV shows about mental illness like never before; they talk about mental illness in a newfound language; and they think they are the craziest people on earth.

And indeed all this drug taking is a profoundly, even outrageously, American phenomenon. Americans adore their prescription drugs like no other people on earth, but they really, really adore their psychiatric drugs. Americans are responsible for almost half of the world's prescription drug sales,[47] but the disparity is even greater when it comes to CNS (central nervous system) agents. In 2006, about two-thirds of the money spent on antidepressants was accounted for by the United States.[48] And in 2003 approximately 83 percent of the global market for attention deficit hyperactivity disorder medications was accounted for by the United States, and mainly by U.S. children.[49]

There of course has forever been a war within the American character between Puritanism and excess, with the pendulum swinging often violently between the two poles. It wasn't long ago that Americans were accused, by Peter Kramer, in a passage from *Listening to Prozac*, of "pharmacological Calvinism": "Study after study has shown that, when it comes to prescribed drugs, Americans are conservative. Doctors tend to underprescribe relative to the recommendations of academic psychiatrists for mental conditions, and patients tend to take less medicine than doctors prescribe . . . Relative to the practice in other industrialized countries, prescribing in the United States is moderate."[50] What was true in 1993, according to Kramer, is a distant and faded, even laughable, memory. The pendulum has swung so far the other way that it is hard to fathom that Kramer's statement could actually have been made just a decade and a half ago. Pharmacological Calvinism has turned into pharmacological Caligula.

This is not to say that mental illness isn't, in essence, a product of problematic neurotransmitters and faulty brain functioning—the evidence is overwhelming that it is—and that these drugs aren't extraordinarily effective at times for the people they were developed for, people with severe psychiatric conditions. It is and they are. I have witnessed the lifesaving impact of the drugs for people who really need them, people with true medical illnesses like schizophrenia, bipolar disorder, and major depression. Many of the severely ill clients that I worked with would not have survived without the drugs. But in our characteristic American impatience and zeal, the drugs have been hyped beyond the limits of their ability to help most people; their efficacy with specific populations has been overgeneralized and misapplied to treat the troubles of the masses generally and upper-middle-class angst specifically; their largely unknown mechanisms of action have been made, literally, into cartoons; and their subtleties have been ignored and side effects overlooked.

While in recent years some individual European countries have used antidepressants at rates even higher than the United States, all this psychiatric drug-taking remains a largely American phenomenon. The drugs were largely invented here; most of the big drug companies are here; the American citizenry has typically been the "early adopters" of these drugs; and the drugs have been marketed here like no where else on earth. Americans have the most luridly expensive urine in the world.

CHAPTER TWO

The Commerce of Mood

Over most of the last fifteen years, Big Pharma—or the medico-pharmaceutical complex, as it is sometimes called—has ranked first or at the very top on all three of *Fortune*'s profitability measures. Starting about 1980, drug companies, which barely existed before World War II, have been the toast of Wall Street.[1] In 2002, the combined profits of the top ten drug companies were greater than the profits *of all the other 490 Fortune 500 companies put together.*[2] In 2001, Merck reaped more than $7 billion in profits, and Pfizer $12 billion in 2003.[3] Put another way: the $7 billion of profits Pfizer amassed in 2001 was greater than the Fortune 500 profits in the home building, apparel, railroad, and publishing industries combined. Merck's profits that year exceeded the combined profits of the Fortune 500–listed semiconductor, pipeline, food production, crude oil production, hotel, casino, and resort industries.[4] The compensation given to the top executives is equally transcendent. William C. Steere Jr., Pfizer's chairman, made $40 million in 2000 as Pfizer's chairman. But that paled in comparisin to his unexercised stock options of $130 million. Which was nothing compared to the stock options held by the CEO of Bristol–Myers Squibb, which amounted to $227 million. And it's not just the CEOs: in 2000, the average unexercised stock options of the top executives at Merck were $73 million; at Bristol–Myers Squibb, $65 million; at Pfizer, $54 million; at Eli Lilly, $33 million.[5]

Even after the woes that Big Pharma experienced between 2004 and 2007—the withdrawal of Vioxx from the market, the loss of large portions of the injectable flu vaccines because of quality control problems, and a growing public awareness of profiteering and an all-too-cozy relationship with the Bush administration—no one should worry unduly about the industry's fortunes. The Bush administration has had very close ties with the drug industry: Donald Rumsfeld, for example, was formerly CEO of Searle, which was acquired by Pharmacia, the makers of Xanax, and budget director Mitch Daniels was vice president of Eli Lilly.

For all the talk of disaster, the top seven U.S.-based drug companies made $34 billion profit from $193 billion in revenues in 2004, which translates to an 18 percent profit margin.[6] In 2006, the return on revenues for the pharmaceutical industry was 20 percent, making it the second most profitable industry in America.[7] By contrast, the profit margin of the construction industry was 2 percent and the automotive industry 1 percent. As is typically the case, these companies made more profit than they spent on research and development. It's only in the pharmaceutical or the oil industries that a 20 percent profit margin would be considered a slump. Kurt Vonnegut identified an enduring truth when he wrote in *Cat's Cradle*: "The hand that stocks the drug stores rules the world."

What is not so widely known is that, as a group, psychotherapeutic drugs, along with cardiovascular medications, have been the primary source of Big Pharma's profits over the last two decades. Collectively, central nervous system drugs, of which psychiatric drugs are the primary component, are among the fastest-growing segments of the world market. CNS diseases, which include Alzheimer's and Parkinson's as well as psychiatric diseases, are, well, hot. They represent dream marketing opportunities for drug makers, for a number of reasons. Psychiatric and neurological diseases tend to be chronic, meaning that those who truly suffer from them will, or should, take the medications for the rest of their lives. CNS diseases also tend to be serious, requiring high rates of hospitalization, and, according to industry analysts, they are on the rise, given the growing aged population and "the physiological/psychological stress of current lifestyles."[8] Carl Elliott, physician, bioethicist, and author of *Better Than Well: American Medicine Meets the American Dream*, wrote in 2003: "The pharmaceutical industry is now the most profitable industry in America, with 18 percent annual profit margins, and its most profitable class of product is the antidepressant drugs."[9] Which would mean that antidepressants have been the most profitable product in the most profitable industry in the most profitable country in the world.

Psychiatric drugs are the number-one therapeutic category among the world's top two hundred prescription medicines.[10] In 2006, antidepressants were the sixth best-selling category of drugs in the world, and antipsychotics were the seventh best-selling.[11] The antipsychotic Zyprexa, the seventh best-selling drug in the world in 2005, was responsible for 30 percent of Lilly's revenues that year.[12] Effexor accounted for 18 percent of Wyeth's revenues in 2005.[13] The antipsychotic Risperdal was Johnson & Johnson's second best-selling drug in 2004. And in 2004, the psychiatric drugs Zoloft, Seroquel, Celexa, and Lexapro were each the number-one or the number-two best-selling products of their respective manufacturers.[14]

If one were to put the most brilliant drug marketers in the world in a room for a month, they would not be able to come up with a more propitious set of contingencies upon which to launch a new category of drugs than that Prozac enjoyed by the time of its 1988 introduction. Its timing was perfect for two reasons: first, when antidepressants came along in the late 1980s and 1990s, they matched what Americans were looking for in their drugs; and second, their appearance coincided with the era when big drug companies were transforming themselves from merely profitable companies to the toast of Wall Street.

For all the puritanical condemnations of licit and illicit

substances—the self-righteous, simplistic "Just Say No" campaigns and the other-directed War on Drugs (in which we place the blame for our mass consumption of cocaine not on ourselves but on the Colombians and Venezuelans)—Americans have never been able to get by for very long without their drugs. Prohibition was a disaster and lasted only a little more than a decade. Each new generation of Americans either chooses a favorite drug or creates one: marijuana and LSD and speed in the '60s and '70s, PCP and crack in the '80s, ecstasy and crystal meth in recent years. Alcohol is of course the constant. The War on Drugs will likely never be won because Americans don't want it to be won. But even within that context of the ongoing love affair of Americans with their substances, the SSRI phenomenon has been exceptional in the rapidity of its penetration into the masses.

Prozac was blessed by having a great opening act: Valium. Valium did what all great opening acts are supposed to do—set the stage, pave the way, and make the main event shine. Introduced in 1963 after being developed by the legendary Dr. Leo Sternbach of Hoffman–La Roche, Inc., Valium was one of the benzodiazepines, quick-acting antianxiety drugs which are, in effect, minor tranquilizers. Sternbach, who died in 2005 at the age of ninety-seven, was a kind of genius pharmacologist who also invented the sleeping pill Dalmane, the antiseizure medication Klonopin, and Arfonad, which limits bleeding during brain surgery. He held 241 drug patents by the end of his career.[15] Far and away his most famous creation, though, was Valium—which he tested on himself only to discover that it made him depressed.[16]

Six years after its introduction, Valium became the most common drug in America. It remained so until 1982. In 1978, at the peak of its popularity, 2.3 billion pills were sold. Valium became so popular in the corporate world that it was known as "Executive Excedrin."[17] In the 1960s and 1970s, Valium became a clinical and cultural phenomenon that presaged—though never rivaled—the Prozac Nation '90s. The Rolling Stones had a hit song, "Mother's Little Helper," about the use of pills by stressed-out housewives ("She goes running for the shelter of her mother's little helper, and it helps her on her way, gets her through her busy day"), and Valium pills were the "dolls" in Jacqueline Susann's over-the-top 1966 best seller *Valley of the Dolls.* The success of Valium was so impressive that Eli Lilly initially considered marketing Prozac as an antianxiety agent.[18]

It wasn't until later that an unanticipated tragic flaw to Valium emerged. The pills were highly addictive when they weren't supposed to be. Despite initial claims that the drug had neither addiction potential nor caused a withdrawal syndrome, anecdotal and then scientific evidence soon suggested otherwise.[19] Valium makes one feel very good very quickly, in less than an hour. The relaxing sensations are wonderful and soothing. They are also tremendously addictive, physically and psychologically. Anybody experienced in working with addictions will tell you that "benzo addiction" is particularly difficult and painful to overcome, often requiring lengthy inpatient treatment to address. (I have spoken to many addicts who have said that benzos are the most difficult of all drugs to kick.) As word of Valium's addictiveness spread, the stigma associated with the drug grew rapidly. Comedian Rodney Dangerfield said he took it daily along with 136 other pills. Reagan adviser Michael Deaver attributed his deceit before a federal grand jury to the influence of a Valium haze. The stigma often took the form of suspicions of feminine weakness. (As with the SSRIs, women took Valium at twice the rate of men.) Elizabeth Taylor acknowledged a steady diet of Valium and Jack Daniel's, and Tammy Faye Bakker, televangelist Jim Bakker's wife, admitted her addiction to Valium, which she took—very inventively, I might add—by means of a nasal spray solution. In response to such revelations, the U.S. Senate conducted hearings on tranquilizer addiction in 1979.[20] And as quickly as Valium rose, it fell. Sales plummeted in the early 1980s. Valium is now the forty-first most prescribed generic drug in America.[21]

The profound and lasting historical legacy of Valium is that it brought psychiatric drugs into the mainstream. Unlike earlier drugs, such as Haldol, Thorazine, and lithium, which were taken exclusively by the denizens of loony bins, Valium was taken by just about everybody—by the "worried well," the "functioning." Everybody—

housewives and judges, salesmen and politicians—took Valium. For the first time in history, it was *okay* to take psychiatric drugs. Simply put, you didn't have to be crazy—*that is, you didn't have to be mentally ill*—to take the pills. This was a sea change, an immensely profound paradigm shift in thinking about psychiatric drugs.

On a broader societal level, when the SSRIs arrived in 1988, they delivered exactly the things that Americans wanted and expected in their drugs.

Over the course of the 1980s, the United States was, on so many fronts, "on the rebound," attempting to sober up from the excesses and eccentricities of the immediately preceding decades. On the drug front, there was a collective revulsion against the psychedelic experimentation of the 1960s, the marijuana clouds of the 1970s, the cocaine-fueled excesses of the early 1980s. By the late 1980s, mainstream America had had enough of cocaine in the bathroom at yuppie parties, of LSD in college, of marijuana in the suburbs, and certainly, of heroin and crack in the streets. There was a particular revulsion against intravenous street drugs, and the new plague, HIV and AIDS, associated with them. Crack became particularly notorious, as tales of its addictiveness and human devastation—"crack babies" and sunken-eyed, spindly "crack whores"—spread. In society at large, epitomized by Ronald Reagan and the Reagan Revolution, there was a parallel desire to "get straight," to get America "back on track." The long hair of the 1960s and 1970s was replaced by "short back and sides," and the overall scruffiness, cynicism, and eccentricities of earlier decades were replaced by aerobics, patriotism, yuppie ambition, and a new selfish, and self-absorbed, arrogance and swagger. There was a new pressure to perform, *to function*. A great deal of this emanated from a growing awareness of the new economic realties: in particular, a prevailing awareness especially on the part of younger Americans that cyclical recession had become a permanent feature of the economic landscape; that a college education in and of itself no longer guaranteed much security; and a creeping, damaging awareness that theirs was the first generation in American history likely to do less well than their parents. No longer was the emphasis for young people on escape, spiritual exploration, and hedonistic self-fulfillment, but on competitive self-improvement, both individually and nationally. It was "CleanUp Time," as a John Lennon song of 1980 was called.

That ability to function and the capacity to achieve were exactly what Prozac delivered,[22] or at least that's what the marketers said. (And indeed that's how psychiatric disorders are ultimately defined—if you look at the *Diagnostic and Statistical Manual of Mental Disorders* (DSM), the American Psychiatric Association's diagnostic manual, the decisive and clinching feature of most psychiatric disorders is the inability to function in occupational and social settings.) Prozac, Ritalin, etc. promised to help you do what you needed to do—pay attention in school (when prescribed for attention deficit hyperactivity disorder), help you focus on the important things (when prescribed for obsessive-compulsive disorder), get to work on time (when prescribed for insomnia), make you happier and more fun to be around (when prescribed for depression), help you settle down (when prescribed for generalized anxiety disorder), make you socially adequate, and perhaps even suave and wonderfully self-possessed (when prescribed for social anxiety disorder), make you less scared of snakes and heights and airplanes (when prescribed for phobias), and help a man have satisfactory sex (when prescribed for premature ejaculation). As the Harvard political scientist Harvey Mansfield has written, "Ritalin tempers the high spirits of boys, and Prozac raises the low spirits of women"—so both can be closer to the socially acceptable norm.[23] By contrast, the drugs of the 1960s and 1970s were meant to deliver the opposite: they were not intended for functioning, but for doing as little as possible. One took the drugs to loaf, to exit, and to escape. (As the mantra of the day went, "Turn On, Tune In, Drop Out.") The purpose of LSD and marijuana was to get as far away as possible from mundane draggy reality. Taking them, one was choosing not to engage in and, least of all, succeed at the dreary and corrupt affairs of the world.

The other way the SSRIs matched the spirit of their times is in the manner in which they offered individualized solutions (or the promise of an individualized solution) to our problems, at a time when Americans were giving up on collective solutions to social difficulties. Even a decade or two before, an epidemic of depression might have been approached at some sort of societal, government collective fashion. By the 1980s, Americans no longer believed, for the most part, in social programs. Welfare mothers and the like were so successfully vilified by Reagan that politicians could no longer publicly support such programs and get elected. The era of governmental solutions to national problems and challenges (Social Security, the GI Bill, the Great Society, the Space Program) that began with the New Deal ended—if not in reality, at least ideologically—with Reagan. The individual, the self, religion, and the family unit (leading to the 1990s ideological issue of "family values") were again paramount. And of course the 1980s also saw a renewal of the old American theme (or myth) of rugged individualism: Reagan on his horse, Oliver North going haywire, Rambo taking on an entire army.

In perfect accord with these trends, the SSRIs offered nothing if not an individualized treatment for one's problems. Everything about them was solitary. You filled the prescription alone, you took the medications by yourself, you dealt with your insurance plan alone, and you monitored the effects of the medication, usually, alone. As more people took SSRIs, fewer people chose therapy—which, among other things, is mental health treatment in the company of another person. The prevailing paradigm shifted violently. No longer were patients working with a therapist to address their problems; they were working largely alone and in relation only with a pill. The participation of the doctor—once he or she was done with the hasty writing of the prescription—was marginal.

One can just imagine Lyndon Johnson earnestly making one of the goals of his Great Society the raising of the collective morale and spirits of the American public. In earlier days, some sort of collective social program would have been invented to deal with our downward spiral. And that was partially what John F. Kennedy was trying to do with the signing of the Community Mental Health Act of 1963, intended to create a network of outpatient clinics to serve former hospital patients. The drugs of the 1960s were—at least initially, during the earnest and naïve early days of the peace and protest and civil rights movements—ingested in some kind of en masse effort to enhance the spiritual consciousness of the youth who took them. For the most part, people took acid and smoked pot together, sharing the experience, for good or ill, as a collective unit.

The last critical factor—and here the SSRIs influenced the change as much as they were affected by the change—was that the new drugs arrived at just about the time the big drug companies were pursuing marketing and profitability above all other concerns. In other words, the antidepressants came along at the moment when the drug industry was transforming itself into Big Pharma. In the 1970s and 1980s, the profitability of Fortune 500 drug companies was double the median for all industries in the Fortune 500. In the 1990s, the drug industry's profitability grew to almost four times the median for all industries in the Fortune 500. By the early 2000s, it had increased to more than eight times the median.[24]

At this point, the sins of the big drug companies are well known, or at least better known. The excesses and ethical lapses have become so blatant that even mainstream bastions of free enterprise such as *Forbes* have labeled the drug companies as corporate "pill pushers" and accused them of abandoning science for sales.[25]

Drugs are the fastest-growing component in health care, where costs have soared generally.[26] Prices of the best-selling drugs routinely go up at two to three times the rate of inflation. Uninsured patients in the United States pay more for drugs than people who are insured, who have the large HMOs to bargain for them. The United States is unique among Western countries in that it does not limit drug costs in some way.[27] Big Pharma has the largest lobbying contingent in the country—there are more drug lobbyists than members of Congress[28]—which has helped create an extraordinarily regulation-friendly environment for the industry. *The New York Times* has stated baldly that the pharmaceutical industry "often gets what it asks for from Congress and the executive branch."[29] For example, through such lobbying efforts, the length of the patent life of brand-name drugs—that is, the period when the rights to (and profits from) the drugs are exclusively owned by the company that developed them—increased from around eight years in 1980 to about fourteen years in 2000. The extension of those patent lives has been critical to the industry, leading to untold billions of dollars in additional profits.[30]

Where to begin? How does one count the ways?

The natural place to start is the Food and Drug Administration (FDA), which under the Bush administration appears to have perceived itself as being a client of Big Pharma rather than serving the American public.

The FDA is part of the Department of Health and Human Services (HHS), which itself is part of the executive branch of the government, reporting to the president of the United States. The FDA regulates, or is supposed to regulate, the industries that make up, remarkably, almost one-quarter of the American economy.[31]

At the heart of the problem is a curious law, the Prescription Drug User Fee Act (PDUFA), the fourth version of which was submitted for approval to Congress in 2007. The original PDUFA passed in 1992, and it was reauthorized twice, in 1997 and 2002. The intent of the PDUFA was to speed up the time it took for drugs to be approved, and it has certainly done so. Former FDA official Dr. Janet Woodcock, who was director of FDA's Center for Drug Evaluation and Research, has stated that tight deadlines for drug approval were creating "a sweatshop mentality" within the agency.[32]

The mechanism for speeding things up is very simple: the drug companies pay the FDA directly to evaluate and approve their drugs, to the tune of millions of dollars. Under the terms of the current PDUFA, Big Pharma paid the FDA $305 million in 2007 to review their drugs on an expedited basis. Under the proposed PDUFA IV, the annual user fees will be increased to about $393 million. These figures account for *almost 20 percent of the FDA's entire budget and about half of the budget for reviewing drugs.*[33, 34] Part of that money would cover the moving fees and rent for a new facility in Silver Spring, Maryland. If the proposed PDUFA is approved, Big Pharma will literally be paying the FDA's rent![35]

Clearly, objectivity is severely compromised when the fox is minding the henhouse. "The problem is a system in which businesses have control over the evaluation of their own products," Marcia Angell, former editor of *The New England Journal of Medicine*, has said.[36] While the PDUFA structure goes back to the beginning of the Clinton administration, the influence of Big Pharma over the FDA has increased since 2000. "Business has taken a much higher profile at the FDA because of the current administration," Mary Faith Marshall of the University of Minnesota Medical School contends. "There's a much friendlier attitude toward Big Pharma and less emphasis on human subject protection."[37]

The FDA has also been without a permanent commissioner for about half the time that George W. Bush has been in office. In Bush's first term, the FDA was without a permanent commissioner for about 36 months. In Bush's second term, Lester M. Crawford was driven out of office after two months as permanent commissioner for lying to Congress about financial improprieties while he was acting commissioner, specifically the fact that he held stock in companies that the FDA was evaluating. There have also been a high number of temporary appointees managing its centers, including the offices that test the safety and efficacy of drugs. The instability is a stark contrast to the tenure of Dr. David Kessler, who served seven very active years (taking on Big Tobacco) under presidents George H. W. Bush and Bill Clinton. It would seem the answer to this is to fund the FDA adequately and solely with public funds, which were what funded the agency entirely from its founding in 1906 (by Teddy Roosevelt, who was outraged by the conditions described in Upton Sinclair's *The Jungle*) until the advent of the PDUFA.

Some observers feel that the vacancies at the top have been deliberate. Paul Light, a New York University professor who works with the Brookings Institution, said, "There are some in the administration and in the industry who would rather have vacancies at FDA than an aggressive regulator. The theory is that it is better to have no one there than someone who favors a proactive stance that might slow down the industry or raise hard questions about profitable drugs."[38] Despite all this, White House chief of staff Andrew Card said in 2004 (in the wake of the Vioxx scandal, no less) that the FDA was doing a "spectacular job."[39]

Given both a lack of resources and the fact that what resources it has are under political influence, the FDA's power to regulate the drug industry is surprisingly limited. For example, the agency reviews only a small percentage of the drug commercials that air on television. The FDA says, quite rightly, it doesn't have the resources to review the 54,000 drug promotions a year that come its way.[40] The FDA's drug-marketing enforcement arm has only forty employees.[41] Ads do not have to be reviewed and approved before they are aired. "A company could blanket the airwaves with ads for forty-five days before the FDA finishes its review. Even if the ads are pulled, a lot of folks will now be asking their doctor for that drug, which could have risks that weren't fully explained," says Bill Vaughan, a senior policy analyst for Consumers Union, which publishes *Consumer Reports*.[42]

Beyond that, the FDA lacks the capacity to actually fine companies for marketing abuses. All the FDA can do is send warning letters. The first type of letter, an "untitled letter," essentially says "shame on you," and stop running the ads. The consequences are so trivial that some industry executives say, "If you're not getting them, you're not pushing the envelope far enough," according to Mary Pendergast, a former FDA official. The second type of letter, a "warning letter," requires the drug companies only to stop the original ads and issue new ones that correct previous misinformation.[43]

There is a dire need for an objective, scientific evaluation of drug safety. One of every five drugs introduced to the market between 1975 and 2000 was taken off the market, or had to have so-called black box warnings, because of safety concerns.[44] ("Black box warnings," so called because the warning is printed inside a black frame on the package, indicate that the drug may have serious and even life-threatening effects. They are the most serious admonitions that the FDA places on the labels of prescription medications.) "We have been dependent on the pharmaceutical industry to provide the answers," said Dr. Thomas Insel, director of the National Institute of Mental Health. "The questions they want answered are different than the public health questions."[45]

It is also disconcerting that many FDA standards for clinical studies are surprisingly flimsy. The FDA allows studies to recruit what are called "samples of convenience," the result of which is that often patients in studies bear little resemblance to those who will actually take the drug once it is on the market.[46] "Samples of convenience" typically means those patients who are relatively easy to recruit—college students are the classic example. People with severe and persistent mental illness are of course difficult to recruit. As a result, the drugs used to treat severe mental illness have historically rarely been tested on people who actually suffer from extremely severe psychiatric conditions.[47] (To be fair, the industry has modified its approach in recent years and is now actually testing the drugs on people who have the conditions that the drugs are supposed to treat.)[48] Furthermore, most FDA studies of psychiatric drugs need last for only six to eight weeks. This is bizarre and arbitrary, as some psychiatric drugs need a month or longer to take effect, and most psychiatric illnesses, of course, are long-term, if not chronic. (In response to these concerns, the FDA for a brief period in 2005 called on the industry to submit both short-term [six to eight weeks] and long-term [greater than six months] efficacy data on new drugs. This policy, however, was reversed by a unanimous 12–0 vote by an FDA advisory panel, which heard testimony by a coalition of ten drug companies asking them to overturn it.)[49]

The FDA allows clinical trials to be conducted in other countries. The *Asia Times* reports that India has emerged as "a preferred destination for outsourcing clinical trials."[50] An Indian medical journal complains that the country is becoming "the greatest source of human guinea pigs for the global drug industry."[51] GlaxoSmithKline, Eli Lilly, Pfizer, and Novartis all run trials there. Why? Vast numbers of potential research subjects, cheaper costs, and the fact that the patient population is "treatment naïve"—they are largely unexposed to drugs, which makes the evaluation of the effect of a given drug easier. India's other advantages include English-speaking medical personnel, lots of hospitals (700,000 specialty beds), and medical colleges (221). But of all these, cost savings is the big one. Forty percent of the costs of developing a drug come from clinical trials, and India can conduct them for about a third less.[52]

In 2006, the Union of Concerned Scientists surveyed scientists who work at the FDA for their thoughts on what could best be done to improve the integrity of the agency. Almost one thousand responded. The results, which are posted, unedited, on www.ucsusa.org, are revelatory. While there is the occasional "happy camper" who feels that all is right with the world and the occasional response that calls for more Hawaiian shirt days, the overwhelming sentiment is one of poor morale, frustration, and an agency staggering from the influence of politics over science. It is a situation that appears to have gotten significantly worse under the administration of George W. Bush. Some samples from different responses:

> Those who get ahead do so by being yes-men, and by copying and pasting what the drug companies say directly into their reviews. The FDA is presently being stacked at every management level including the lowest levels based on those who will support the big companies' agenda, and the implications for safety and efficacy will be felt long into the future . . . There's also favoritism toward the largest companies, senior management wants us to meet with large companies over minor issues that these companies use to tie us up for months . . . Computer simulations using clearly erroneous models have been used to approve drugs for political reasons.

> When I go to meetings with my upper management, I honestly prepare myself as though I were going to a meeting with an industry representative. Whenever safety or efficacy concerns are raised on scientific grounds . . . these concerns are not taken

> seriously. There is a remarkable amount of pressure placed on reviewers to find "creative" ways to approve problematic drugs. Reviewers who approve drugs consistently get special project-related awards, while those who do an excellent job on a product that doesn't get approved are very clearly ignored.
>
> FDA considers their customer to be the manufacturers. The customer should be the public.
>
> Management should never tell scientists what conclusions would be acceptable.
>
> We need a full-time, permanent commissioner who is not a political appointee. We have not had one in years.

The FDA has not always been so toothless. The agency once had a long and proud tradition of enforcement. On the occasion of the FDA's centennial in 2006, the executive director of the Center for Science in the Public Interest, Michael F. Jacobson, said, "The FDA's centennial is not so much a time to celebrate, but to mourn the FDA's gradual descent into irrelevancy . . . the great Republican president Theodore Roosevelt would be sick to his stomach if he could see how Harvey Wiley's [first FDA commissioner] hard-charging tiger of an agency became such a pliant pussycat." And Representative Henry A. Waxman, Democrat of California, added: "[The] FDA was our country's first consumer protection agency, and Americans have relied on FDA to ensure the safety of their food and drugs for one hundred years. Under the Bush administration, FDA has undermined enforcement and betrayed its consumer-first legacy. FDA must start enforcing the law and return to a culture that places public health concerns ahead of industry profits."[53]

In the drug industry generally, marketing dominates science. The drug companies consistently spend almost double on marketing what they do on research.[54] As omnipresent as drug ads on TV have become, expenditures on advertising make up only a very small portion of the marketing budget. Up to 90 percent of the marketing budgets go directly to manipulating the source—directly toward influencing the doctors themselves—in the form of drug samples, lecture fees, and "educational" grants.[55] The industry spends an unholy $22 billion a year to market directly to doctors, which is the equivalent of about $25,000 per physician per year.[56] To influence hearts and minds, Big Pharma has assembled an army of about one hundred thousand drug sales representatives, called detailers, whose job it is to push product directly to the MDs.[57] The number of detailers has almost tripled in the last ten years, as did the spending on marketing directly to doctors over roughly the same period.[58] "Unbeknownst to most doctors," writes the advocacy group the Center for Policy Alternatives, "drug detailers have access to prescriber reports that let them know—right down to the pill—if their sales pitches are successful. Prescriber reports are weekly lists of every prescription written by every physician, excluding patients' names. Data mining companies like Dendrite International, Verispan, and IMS Health buy this information from pharmacies, pharmacy benefits managers, and insurance companies. Dendrite, for example, purchases information on 150 million prescriptions every month and currently has a database of 5 billion prescriptions. This data is sold to pharmaceutical manufacturers, who distribute doctor-by-doctor prescriber reports to their detailers. Prescriber reports allow detailers to target doctors and adjust sales pitches until they find the ones that work best. Such an invasion of privacy provides no benefit to doctors or patients—it serves only to enrich drug companies and detailers."[59]

Drug companies pay for most of "continuing medical education" programs (in my experience, often thinly disguised as advertising for particular drugs) for doctors, and pay for most medical conferences.[60] First-class airfare, four-star hotels, prizes and giveaways, Sunbelt resort stays, and sumptuous meals are commonplace for presenters. Any casual attendee simply passing through the exhibit spaces can grab enough Zoloft pens, Viagra calendars, and Zyprexa coffee cups to last a decade. Major international conferences, such as the World Congress of Biological Psychiatry, feature bizarre installations to promote the drugs. At the Berlin conference in 2001, Eli Lilly set up what were described as "fun houses" to draw the attention of physicians to their products. In one fun house, called "Prozac," a huge mouselike creature sat in front of a blank TV screen. A confused psychiatrist asked the Lilly reps for clarification and was informed that the mouse represented a depressed man who needed Prozac. Another fun house, "Zyprexa," featured a mirrored room with dozens of telephones hanging from the ceiling. This, the sales reps explained, was an illustration of the communication problems associated with schizophrenia.[61]

To boost the image of the products they sell, drug representatives are typically vivacious and cute and female. "There's a saying that you'll never meet an ugly drug rep," said Dr. Thomas Carli, of the University of Michigan.[62] "Many give off a kind of glow, as if they had just emerged from a spa or salon. And they are always, hands down, the best-dressed people in the hospital," writes Carl Elliott, longtime observer of the drug industry.[63] A common practice is to recruit future drug salespeople from the cheerleading ranks of major colleges. "Pharma Babes," they're called by doctors behind closed doors. T. Lynn Williamson, a "cheering advisor" at the University of Kentucky, says he regularly gets calls from recruiters looking to hire women from his ranks as drug sales representatives. "They watch to see who's graduating. They don't ask what the major is," Williamson says.[64] When I was working in homeless shelters, I was shocked that these bubbly and perky drug reps (all women) would brave our gothic, cavernous, and squalid facilities for even two minutes with the psychiatrist who prescribed the drugs. My clients—most of whom hadn't been in such proximity to an attractive woman for decades—would eye them with a combination of caution, fear, and lust.

If the drug companies spent more money on research instead of marketing, they would avoid their largest current dilemma—their increasing inability to produce good new products. The real problem for Big Pharma is not declining profit margins or loss of political clout—although the Democratic victories in late 2006 sent shockwaves through the industry, for fear that the government would negotiate lower prices of drugs for Medicare. The real concern is the lack of new and innovative drugs. Only twenty new drugs were approved by the FDA in 2005, as compared to fifty-three in 1996.[65] The "pipeline problem," as it is called, speaks to the serious lack of creativity on the part of the industry. Many of the new drugs are actually developed not at the big drug companies but at universities, small biotech firms, and the National Institutes of Health. Big Pharma has instead cast its lot with the pharmaceutical equivalent of picking low-hanging fruit. In recent years, the industry giants have largely gone in for producing what are called "me-too" drugs, slight variants on existing blockbuster medications, rather than searching for something truly new.[66]

While suffering from a lack of innovation in creating new products, the industry has been highly creative, to the point at times of criminal investigation, in pushing the boundaries of their existing products. Major drug companies have been in the news for blatant violations. Under a marketing campaign called "Viva Zyprexa," Eli Lilly pushed Zyprexa, indicated for bipolar and schizophrenia, on patients who did not suffer from either condition. The patients were actually suffering from dementia, a condition for which Zyprexa is not approved. In fact its use for dementia is warned against by the FDA, which has stated that Zyprexa can increase the risk of death for older patients with dementia-related psychosis.[67] In the last few years, Lilly has paid $1.2 billion to settle claims for patients who said they developed diabetes or other diseases after taking the drug.[68] Diabetes is a possible side effect of Zyprexa, according to the American Diabetes Association.[69] (Lilly denied that a link between Zyprexa and diabetes has been proven.[70] In 2007, however, Lilly added strong warnings to Zyprexa's label, indicating the drug's tendency to cause weight gain, high blood sugar, and high cholesterol.)[71] The company has been under federal and state investigation for its marketing practices for Zyprexa.

Lilly is not alone. Almost every major drug company is being investigated criminally or civilly for alleged efforts to promote their drugs beyond their approved uses.[72] Indeed, in 2004, Warner-Lambert, whose parent company is Pfizer, was ordered by the Department of Justice to pay more than $430 million to resolve criminal charges and civil liabilities for its "illegal and fraudulent promotion" for unapproved uses for Neurontin, a popular drug that was approved by the FDA solely as a supplementary drug for epilepsy patients. Instead, Warner-Lambert aggressively marketed the drug for bipolar disorder, various pain disorders, Lou Gehrig's disease (amyotrophic lateral sclerosis), attention deficit disorder, migraine, seizures resulting from drug and alcohol withdrawal, restless-leg syndrome, and as a first-line, single treatment for epilepsy. Among the tactics employed by Warner-Lambert were false claims about Neurontin's efficacy and its approval for off-label uses. According to the Department of Justice, "medical liaisons" were hired who "represented themselves (often falsely) as scientific experts in a particular disease." To promote off-label uses of Neurontin, Warner-Lambert also paid doctors to attend expensive dinners and events, such as trips to Hawaii, Florida, and the Atlanta Olympics. The investigation of Warner-Lambert was initiated by a Dr. David P. Franklin, a former medical liaison himself, who filed a whistleblower action with the federal government. For his services, Dr. Franklin received $24 million, his share of the civil settlement.[73]

By 2000, about two-thirds of biomedical research was funded by the industry and about a third by the government. In 1980, it was the reverse. Of the eighty thousand clinical trials conducted in the United States in a typical year, fifty thousand to sixty thousand are industry-sponsored.[74] An analysis of all clinical trials published in four of the most prestigious psychiatric journals—397 trials—found that 60 percent had received funding from a pharmaceutical company or other interested party. About half of those studies were authored by at least one person with a reported financial conflict of interest. To no one's evident surprise, trials that reported such a conflict of interest were *almost five times more likely* to find positive results about the drug.[75]

For schizophrenia drugs, Lilly, Johnson & Johnson, and other companies have run numerous direct trials, in which their drug is compared with a competing product. All five of the studies paid for by Lilly showed the superiority of their drug Zyprexa to Risperdal, while three of the four Johnson & Johnson studies favored Risperdal over Zyprexa. "The comparative studies are a joke. They are comical. A lot of the scientific literature these days is worthless," says Jack E. Rosenblatt, a psychiatrist.[76] Furthermore, clinical trials that do not favor a company's interest simply do not have to be reported to the FDA. It has been judged that the overreporting of favorable studies has led to a 25 percent overestimate of the effectiveness of antipsychotic drugs, for example. Indeed, the greatest single determinant of an outcome of a published study appears to be whether or not a drug company has sponsored the study.[77]

Sophisticated psychiatrists know to take what they read of a drug in even the best journals with a sizable grain of salt. "Not only is there suspicion of the results that are reported, there's a good chance that what is reported is not generalizable to the people, usually with much more severe problems, that I see day in day out in the clinic," Scott Masters, an assistant professor of clinical psychiatry at Columbia, told me.[78]

So nasty has the business become that drug companies now pay doctors to publish negative things about their competitors' drugs. Trazodone, used often for sleep, is a perfectly good drug. It has been around for a long time, is cheap and effective, and is nonaddictive. The only problem with trazodone is that it is long off-patent, meaning there's comparatively very little revenue left to be generated by its sales. A series of new sleep aids, such as Ambien CR, Lunesta, and Rozerem, have recently tried to move into trazodone's territory. Being new agents, Ambien CR, Rozerem, and Lunesta are at the start of their patent lives and therefore lucrative years. Recently, several articles have been published in the professional journals that have been described as "trazodone-bashing." It turns out that the authors of these articles—university psychiatrists—have been paid by the makers of Ambien, Rozerem, et al. According to *The New York Times*, "a careful reading of these articles reveals a pattern of rhetorical techniques" to put Trazodone in a negative light and downplay its positives.[79]

But the most nefarious and manipulative practice of all is barely known, even within the medical profession. It is a dirty little secret that a good percentage of "scientific" articles in even the top journals are now "ghostwritten"—meaning that a failure to identify, in the author credits, a person who has made substantial contributions to the writing or research of the article. Many journal articles are "ghostwritten to order for drug companies, often by writers for medical communications companies, who appear to be acting as intermediaries to distance drug companies from the articles."[80] Some academics simply put their names on the articles already produced by the pharmaceutical company, while others work from a draft given to them. A Georgetown University medical professor, Dr. Adriane Fugh-Berman, has documented how she was contacted by RxComms, a British medical communications company, to author a review of interactions between herbs and a generic anticoagulant called warfarin.* "Months later, I received a completed 2,848-word draft, with an abstract, references, and a table, ready for submission to a journal, with my name on it. A note asked me to return it with any changes within seven days." Dr. Fugh-Berman declined, but no matter, another "author" was quickly found. RxComms appeared to have been hired by Astrazeneca, who was preparing to release a drug to compete with warfarin. Witnesses for Astrazeneca later strongly denied any involvement before the British House of Commons.[81] The practice of ghostwriting has been called no less than an ornate form of money laundering.[82]

As one would expect, there's good money to be had in ghostwriting. An article published in one of the top journals (e.g., *The New England Journal of Medicine*, *The Lancet*, *The British Medical Journal*) can net the "author" up to $20,000.[83] A 1998 review of articles published in leading journals such as *The Journal of the American Medical Association* and *The New England Journal of Medicine* found that 11 percent were ghostwritten. The fact that authors were paid to write the articles for the drug companies is not disclosed to the reader. Some observers have called

*Warfarin, with its ungainly name, was surely brought to market before the naming of drugs became a sophisticated business.

the 11 percent figure for ghostwritten articles too low.[84] When David Healy and Dinah Cattell investigated the medical literature for all the articles published on Zoloft for the years 1998, 1999, and 2000, they discovered that ghostwritten articles outnumbered authentically authored articles by fifty-five to forty-one. Of course, ghostwritten articles describe a more effective and benign version of Zoloft than the traditionally authored articles. Five of the six ghost-written articles that concerned pediatric psychopharmacology failed to mention that 9 percent of the children in trials experienced suicidal thoughts or took an action toward suicide.[85]

All of which is to say that the industry has invaded the academy, and the academy has only been too happy to let them in. *The New England Journal of Medicine* has a sensible policy requiring its authors to list their financial relationship with the drug companies. The only problem is that the policy can be somewhat impractical. For an article on the antidepressant nefazodone, the authors' financial ties with the makers of the drug were so voluminous that listing them in full would have taken up too much space in the *Journal*. The editors were compelled to merely summarize the financial ties and list them in full on the Web site.[86]

And when it comes to being involved with money from the drug industry, psychiatry in particular is a main offender. "Psychiatrists earn more money from drug companies than doctors in any other specialty," wrote *The New York Times* in reporting a story about lecture fees and gifts given to psychiatrists in Vermont and Minnesota.[87] And more than half of the psychiatrists involved in developing the 1994 edition of the DSM had financial ties to drug companies.[88]

One can argue that financial self-interest is influencing medicine to its core, in the very defining of how to practice medicine. Almost two-thirds of the doctors who frame the formal guidelines of clinical best practice have received funds to conduct research, and more than a third have worked for pharmaceutical companies as employees or as consultants. Seven percent of authors admitted that their relationship with the pharmaceutical industry influenced their writing of guidelines, but 19 percent thought their co-authors were influenced.[89]

The blame here, in my view, ultimately lies with the doctors and the universities, not the big drug companies. For all their tawdry manipulations, the drug companies are only doing what corporations are supposed to do in this system—make a profit at virtually any cost. Unlike the doctors, the drug companies have taken no Hippocratic oath and generally make few claims to act in the public's best interest. Casting ultimate blame on the drug companies is a little like blaming a wolf for attacking a deer.

Here's the problem, in one stroke: Arthur Caplan, director of the University of Pennsylvania Center for Bioethics, has publicly advised doctors not to take gifts from Big Pharma. He self-righteously proclaimed in January 2001: "The more you yield to economics, the more you're falling to a business model that undercuts arguments for professionalism." Sounds good, but there's a problem with Caplan's moral high horse: he himself consults for the drug and biotech industries and runs a center funded in part by Pfizer, AstraZeneca, and Schering-Plough. But no need to worry: as a sign of concern for the influence of industry interests, the American Medical Association has planned a $590,000 program to raise doctors' awareness of the ethical problems of accepting drug industry gifts. The initiative came about as a result of gifts from Pfizer, Lilly, GlaxoSmithKline, AstraZeneca, Bayer, Procter & Gamble, and Wyeth-Ayerst.[90]

While the public, historically, has been innocently unaware of these details, they are starting to get wise. In the public's view, the pharmaceutical industry has recently joined the oil industry as the most exploitative and reviled sector of corporate America. The perception of manipulation and arrogance on the part of Big Pharma is starting to stick. A trust factor appears to have been violated. Between 1996 and 2002, the portion of the public who distrusted information from clinical research professionals shot up, from 28 percent to 75 percent.[91] *The New York Times* noted that by 2005, consumers seemed to be less confident in drug marketing. "A lot of the demand that the industry has created over the years has been through promotion, and for that promotion to be effective, there has to be trust," said Richard Evans, an analyst at Sanford C. Bernstein & Company, an investment research company. "That trust has been lost."[92]

For all the well-documented excesses and the slick distortions, I was most jarred by an ad for Zoloft that made the rounds in 2006 in big-circulation and women's magazines like *Glamour*. (Women's lifestyle magazines are among the favorite venues of the drug companies to advertise to the public.) This ad featured a case study: Cynthia's story, presented with a great deal of specificity. Cynthia, age fifty-seven, lives in Portland, Washington. Long after her divorce from Tom, she continued to feel sad. She saw her doctor, who prescribed Zoloft, and she now feels much, much better. At the top was a little asterisk that at first I missed: "Story not based on actual person." The transparency of the conceit! The duplicity! The subterfuge! I had gotten quite caught up in Cynthia's story and was shocked by the brazenness of the distortion.

But the greatest illustration of the shift to marketing occurred with the August 12, 1997, loosening of regulations by the Food and Drug Administration on direct to consumer (DTC) advertising. Paxil, Zoloft, and the like (as well as Celebrex, Viagra, and Claritin) are now nightly visitors to the homes of millions of Americans by virtue of their ceaseless presence on prime-time television. The actual mechanism that sprang the entire DTC drug advertising industry was bizarrely simple. Starting in 1997, the FDA waived the requirement that drug makers list a detailed summary of a drug's side effects and contraindications in advertising. It became sufficient for companies to cite only a drug's major risks and provide a Web address and toll-free number where consumers could get more information. It was that modest a change in regulations that made advertising on TV possible.[93]

By focusing almost exclusively on the twenty or so "blockbuster" drugs (which are defined by more than $1 billion in annual sales), DTC advertising has strongly increased the sales of a few top drugs at the expense of the others. It has been proven repeatedly that when consumers see the ads, they ask their doctors for those drugs, and more often than not the harried physician writes the prescription despite his or her ambivalence. Doctors accede to the vast majority of prescription requests for drugs that their patients have seen advertised on TV, despite feeling less than confident about the appropriateness of the medication choice half of the time.[94] So burdensome has this become that 8 of 10 doctors surveyed in 2006 favored a moratorium on DTC advertising for new drugs.[95]

One enterprising study arranged for *trained actors* to make appointments with doctors, act as if they were depressed, and then ask the doctor for an antidepressant. When the depressed actors requested a specific brand, doctors wrote a prescription for that brand 50 percent of the time. When the actors asked for any antidepressant, they were given a prescription three-quarters of the time. And when they didn't even ask for a drug, they were given a prescription one-third of the time.[96]

There are other creative (read: manipulative) ways to get the brands directly out to the consumers, doctors be damned. Pfizer has marketed a "value card" for Viagra, offering a free seventh prescription, clearly targeted for men who don't have insurance coverage for the drug. The makers of Ambien have offered a week's worth of their pills for free.[97] "The Lunesta 7-Night Challenge" made the rounds in newspapers and on television in 2007. The print ads exhorted: "Ask your doctor how to get 7 nights of Lunesta absolutely free!"[98]

Paxil and Zoloft in particular have been the recipients of heavy DTC rotations. Paxil's story is a particularly sordid, and successful, episode in the history of drug marketing. Paxil was a late entrant to the SSRI party—not arriving until 1993, five years after Prozac and a year after Zoloft. Sales prospects seemed limited. In response, GlaxoSmithKline positioned Paxil as an antianxiety drug, and on April 16, 2001, got their prize: FDA approval as an agent for "generalized anxiety disorder," previously a little-known condition. GlaxoSmithKline cranked up an aggressive public relations campaign—an amalgam of profiles of generalized anxiety sufferers given out to local news programs, patient surveys meant to inform the populace of the hidden epidemic, expert testimony by eminent psychiatrists, a blizzard of newspaper articles, and, most pointedly, an onslaught of DTC ads on television.[99] As part of an earlier campaign for "social anxiety disorder" ("Imagine Being Allergic to People" was the slogan), GlaxoSmithKline spent $92 million in one year to market Paxil—more than Nike spent to market its top shoes.[100] The result of all this: Paxil passed Prozac and Zoloft and became the world's ninth best-selling drug.[101]

The marketing has been so excessive that the drug companies clearly took advantage of the events of September 11 for sales. Even *Psychiatric News*, a journal of the American Psychiatric Association, said that drug makers like Glaxo found 9/11 "a marketing opportunity." According to Nielsen Media Research, drug ads increased dramatically in the weeks after the attacks. In October 2001 alone, Glaxo spent $16 million on advertising Paxil, almost twice what they spent the previous October.[102] It worked. Medicaid recipients, for example, who lived within three miles of the World Trade Center filed 18 percent more antidepressant prescriptions in the three months after the attacks.[103] Some ads for Paxil appeared after shows depicting the World Trade Center towers collapsing. One television viewer, Rebecca Ames, commented, "The drug companies have to push those drugs, but it does make my little eyebrow go up a bit. The commercials make it seem like if you take the drug, all your troubles will go away."[104]

Perhaps the best of all the television commercials was the Zoloft "dot" series, which was in heavy rotation in the early 2000s. In one of the ads, an animated black-and-white anguished face in the form of a blobby circle is ensconced in a dark cave. "You know when the world seems like a sad and lonely place?" a voiceover says. "You may feel tired, hopeless, and empty inside. You're anxious, and you don't enjoy the things you onced loved," one hears as a colorful butterfly appears. The animation then morphs into two nerve cells with chemicals moving between them. The simultaneously soothing and authoritative voice continues: "Zoloft, a prescription medicine, can help. It works to correct chemical imbalances in the brain, which may be related to symptoms of depression." The face returns, now smiling, and bounces along after the fluttering butterfly. An appealing logo for Zoloft appears, and then the voice intones, "When you know more about what's wrong, you can help make it right."[105]

The genius of the advertisement is that it made the symptoms of depression cute, funny, and accessible. In other words, the exact opposite of what mental turmoil is actually like. Furthermore, when the dread side effects—sexual problems, diarrhea, and nausea—of Zoloft are mentioned in rapid and obligatory fashion, the accompanying image is of the recovered and happy Dot. The happy pictures dominate the harsh information: the image is more powerful than the words that accompany it.[106]

Serious talent was brought to bear on the Dot ad. A famous animator, Patrick Smith, conceived the Dot character, by his own admission, while under the influence of alcohol.[107] The major advertising agency Deutsch Inc. produced the ad. In an interview on CNN, Val DiFebo of Deutsch said of the Dot ad: "What we thought was important here was to have Dot communicate to people how Dot was feeling." Of the Dot ad campaign in general, DiFebo said, "You're going to see them when you wake up in the morning and when you go to bed at night, because we know that's where you are and we want you to see these ads."[108] Dot has had a wide impact. Dot has inspired a "Bouncy, the Zoloft Dot" fan listing on the Web (in which one fan wrote she wished that Dot was available as a stuffed animal) and articles in *The New York Times*. Dot figures in Alison Pace's novel *Pug Hill*, wherein a neurotic New York thirtysomething woman finds one of her greatest sources of comfort to be watching the Zoloft commercial.

The general influence of DTC advertising is such that, when AstraZeneca began a massive media campaign for Nexium—"the purple pill"—for acid reflux disease, a psychiatric emergency room nurse told me that her department was flooded with calls from people who wanted to know how they could get this great new pill and what exactly it could do for them. Pharmacists say that in the days after a news story or a new DTC ad for a medication comes out they observe a massive increase in prescriptions for that medication.[109]

While DTC advertising has attracted much criticism, and talk of bans, Big Pharma's spending on it has only gone up. Indeed, DTC advertising of drugs is illegal everywhere in the world except for the United States and New Zealand.[110] Drugs are now the second most advertised product in America, after automobiles.[111] And whereas the money spent on advertising cars went down in 2006, the money on shilling drugs has gone up.

But even before the TV ads, the marketers of Prozac fundamentally changed how drugs were defined. Before Prozac, the brand names of drugs were generally some simplified version of their scientific and generic names. For example: haloperidol (generic name) became Haldol (brand name). Prozac, the scientific name of which is fluoxetine, was the largest and splashiest psychiatric drug whose public name was specifically created to evoke saleable images and ideas: in this case, the "pro" connoting positivity, and the "zac" the reassurance and exactitude of science.[112] Since Prozac's smashing success, it has become all but de rigueur that new blockbuster drugs have brand names that simultaneously soothe, invigorate, and inspire—the names of Viagra, Celebrex, Claritin, and others have all followed Prozac's lead. In fact, the naming of drugs is now big business. "Coming up with a brand naming used to be an afterthought," says Bill Trombetta, a professor of pharmaceutical marketing. "But today, pharmaceutical companies realize that they need to brand drugs as early as they can and build equity in the brand."[113] The stakes are so high that drug companies now work with branding agencies to select just the right name . . . a name like Zoloft, uplifting and scientific all at the same time. The hard, decisive sounds of the letters *X*, *Z*, *C*, and *D* are attractive to drug namers. According to James L. Detorre, the president of the Institute (which came up with the names for Lipitor, Clarinex, and Allegra), "the harder the tonality of the name the more efficacious the product in the mind of the physician and the end user."[114] The cost of developing a trade name for a drug is an estimated $500,000 to $2.5 million.[115] Names are registered even before the drug exists. There are "only so many *Z*'s and *X*'s to go around," Professor Trombetta notes.[116] The name *Zoloft* was invented by Frank Delano, a legendary marketing guru, who also created the names of Nissan's Pathfinder and Quest minivans, GMC's Yukon, and Primerica Financial Services.[117]

Prozac et al. were among the first drugs to be sold as "lifestyle agents." From their very introduction, Prozac and later antidepressants were defined, brilliantly, not so much as alleviating symptoms of an illness but capable of something far more decisive and fundamental, "existential," if you will—restoring those who consumed them back to their true selves and allowing them to return to the kind of vital, achieving life that it is presumed we all want. Hence the marketing slogans:

Prozac: "Welcome Back."
Paxil: "Your Life Is Waiting."
Wellbutrin: "I'm Ready to Experience Life."
Effexor: "The Change You Deserve"

Prozac made it acceptable for drugs to be, simply and solely, lifestyle agents, paving the way for Viagra (slogan: "Get Back to Mischief") and Cialis ("If a Relaxing Moment Turns Into the Right Moment, Will You Be Ready?"). In being defined as agents of self rather than mediators of illness, the drugs were applicable to a far, far wider audience than merely the seriously depressed—marketable to anyone who wants to "experience life" and to "dream" and feel they "deserve a change," which is, of course, just about all of us.

The excitement and hype surrounding the Serotonin Empire would all be justified if the drugs really worked as well and as straightforwardly as advertised. The problem is that when you dig deeper into the data, more serious and disturbing problems with the drugs emerge.

Retrospective analysis by David Healy, the premier authority on the history of psychiatric drugs, has shown how flimsy the "evidence base" was in the trials that launched the SSRIs. As Healy has written, "There was . . . an extraordinary contrast between the marketing hype and the trials underpinning it."[118] In Zoloft's submission for licensure, only one of the five studies indicated superiority over placebo. For

Prozac, four testing centers showed positive results, and four, negative results. Another group of studies, with extremely positive results for Prozac, was removed at the request of the FDA because the outcomes were at odds with the other data generated.[119] Later, it became clear that a large number of trials with less than favorable results for the SSRIs were simply not reported and that from the very start, suicidal thinking and behavior were associated with the drugs. But in marketing their product, the drug companies did not have to reveal anything about the weak evidence on which their registrations were based.[120]

Second, while the SSRIs have been proven to have real efficacy for many if not most people who suffer from major depression, there is no evidence or only very limited evidence that they work for people with "subsyndromal" depression—that is, people who have one or two of the symptoms of major depression, like insomnia or restlessness, but not the six highly specific criteria that are required to meet the diagnosis. And with the rates of subsyndromal depression outnumbering major depression by two to one,[121] it is mainly these people, if they have any significant symptoms at all, that doctors—particularly primary care doctors, who now prescribe the large majority of antidepressants—are encountering in their offices. Depending on whom you consult, the efficacy of these drugs either goes way down with people with lesser conditions or does not exist at all. Scott Masters, the psychiatrist at Columbia, says, "When I have a patient who is clearly seriously depressed—suicidal, unable to feel any pleasure whatsoever, unable to get out of bed—I can give them an antidepressant and know that it has a seventy or eighty percent chance of being effective. Which is fantastic—that's a greater success rate than most treatments in medicine. But if I have a patient who is just unhappy or fatigued, I have no sense if the medication is going to work. The efficacy clearly goes down in subsyndromal cases."[122] That ineffectiveness and consumer dissatisfaction is reflected in the extraordinarily high rates of early discontinuation of antidepressants. A 2004 study of 27,000 people taking SSRIs revealed that more than a third of patients failed to renew their prescription within thirty days of the end of the initial prescription.[123] Jay

Pomerantz, a Harvard psychiatrist, writes, "Studies clearly show that antidepressants are no more effective than placebo in treating mild depression . . . If what we are seeing is a pattern of widespread antidepressant prescribing for a multitude of subsyndromal, amorphous patient complaints, it suggests that antidepressants have become the modern-day sugar pill."[124] "Doctors should . . . refrain from prescribing unless depression is severe enough," writes the *British Medical Journal.* "Research so far justifies antidepressants only for major depression."[125] Meanwhile, the fact remains that the drugs are just not all that effective for depression in general. Arif Khan, a psychiatrist and researcher in Washington state, used the Freedom of Information Act to obtain the FDA clinical trial database for antidepressant drugs, which included Prozac, Zoloft, Paxil, Serzone, Remeron, Wellbutrin, and Effexor. Khan examined 45 trials, involving about 9,000 patients, and found there was an average symptom reduction of 44 and 48 percent in patients treated with the drugs, and 36 percent with patients treated with placebo after eight weeks of treatment. At the end of the day, an unimpressive difference, unworthy of the hype.[126]

In the absence of data, the American Psychiatric Association simply has no treatment guidelines for the pharmacological treatment of subsyndromal depression. (There are extensive guidelines for major depressive disorder.) The U.S. government's Agency for Health Care Policy and Research, in preparing a report on recommended treatments for depression, reviewed 315 clinical studies evaluating medications and found a grand total of *three* trials on subsyndromal depression worthy of review. Their conclusion: Clinicians who "choose to generalize efficacy data from adult patients with major depression" two other kinds of patients, such as those with subsyndromal depression, or children and adolescents "should do so with care."[127] In the last decade and a half, doctors have clearly *not* used care with antidepressants. "It seems that antidepressants, SSRIs in particular, have replaced benzodiazepines [i.e., Valium, Klonopin, etc.] as the drugs of choice when the physician is at a loss to get the patient out of the office," writes Dr. Pomerantz. With little data and with pressure from managed-care companies reluctant to approve psychotherapy, which they feel is more expensive, doctors have taken it upon themselves to dole out these drugs to patients whose heads are swimming with the latest Paxil ad on TV.

It is important to note, however, that much of the overprescribing is more well-intentioned, or at least naïve or indifferent to the possible consequences, than conspiratorial. As long as there was a chance that the drugs worked (and the vexing and confusing thing is that the drugs do sometimes work in subsyndromal patients) and they were considered safe, what was the harm in giving out these medicines like "sweets," as a British newspaper put it?[128] Before SSRIs were first introduced, the prevalent antidepressants were a class of drug called tricyclics. Tricylics can be fatal when taken in overdose (not a good feature for a drug taken by depressed people), and accordingly, their use was monitored closely by doctors. "Tricyclics were not prescribed like candy. Nobody would write a month's supply of tricyclics and send the patient away," Julio Licinio, a professor of psychiatry at UCLA, recalls.[129] The SSRIs are safe in terms of overdose, which in itself represented a dramatic step forward for antidepressant medication, and it lulled doctors and patients into the false impression that the drugs were safe and largely side-effect free, period.

Initially, this favorable side-effect profile of SSRIs was a key selling point. Peter Kramer, for example, exults about their comparative lack of side effects in *Listening to Prozac.* (To reread *Listening to Prozac* is to realize how dated it is. It has the "gee whiz" infatuation of a first love affair. Nobody writes like that about Prozac anymore!) Also, a close reading reveals that Kramer's evidence base was the stories of about twelve patients. The appeal of the book lies in Kramer's lyrical and winning writing style and intriguing philosophical speculations, rather than any substantive empirical data. Kramer was also misinterpreted. To my reading, Kramer is at least as pro-therapy as he is pro-medication, but, as usual, all the attention went to the drugs.

The rub is that SSRIs are no longer considered as safe as they were initially believed to be. "[E]xperience has shown that some side effects are more common and problematic than initially suspected," said Norman Sussman, director of the psychopharmacology research service at New York University. According to reports, insomnia (experienced by 15 percent to 20 percent of patients), weight gain (experienced by 18 percent to 50 percent), sexual dysfunction, nausea, diarrhea, headache, agitation, lethargy, and fatigue are common.[130] In a study of Zoloft with children and adolescents, 17 of 189 subjects dropped out because of side effects, which included agitation, diarrhea, nausea, vomiting, and anorexia.[131] Sleep disturbance is a particularly nettlesome issue. "There are a lot of data showing that people who sleep poorly are more likely to relapse [with depression] and that suicide risk is higher," Sussman said. Sleep problems also often require additional medication: 22 percent to 34 percent of patients taking SSRIs are also prescribed sedatives or hypnotics. There can also be bizarre sexual side effects—such as "yawning-excitement syndrome," in which patients experience sexual arousal when they yawn, even progressing to orgasm. "This is probably underreported," Dr. Sussman said. Patients often say, 'If you hadn't asked me, I wouldn't have mentioned it.' "[132]

Getting off the drugs is a more formidable, and more problematic, task than was first believed. SSRIs were initially marketed as being dependence- and withdrawal-free; indeed, those qualities, which stood in stark contrast to the benzodiazepines, were a dramatic part of their initial appeal. There has since been a creeping awareness that this was wrong. David Healy contends that the manufacturers knew all along that there were dependence and withdrawal problems with the SSRIs. From the mid-1980s on, Beecham Pharmaceuticals/SmithKline Beecham observed withdrawal problems associated with Paxil and commenced an investigation, which indicated that about half of volunteers taking the drug experienced withdrawal problems, including depression, anxiety, dizziness, nightmares, and overall malaise. SmithKline and other companies appear not to have informed regulators of their findings. Healy also found data from the World Health Organization on patient complaints and withdrawal reactions to Paxil that exceeded the rates of even the benzodiazepines. As Healy writes, "It is now clear that the rates at which withdrawal problems have been reported on [Paxil] exceed the rates at which withdrawal problems have been reported on any other psychotropic drug ever."[133] And all one really had to do all along was ask the patients themselves. In 1999, doctors in the Netherlands asked patients what they thought of the drugs. Thirty percent said they thought antidepressants were addictive.[134] Conventional medical wisdom at the time was that SSRIs were, at best, minimally addictive.

In the last few years, reports have begun to crop up in the professional journals of something called, eerily, "antidepressant discontinuation syndrome." Studies have shown that about 20 percent of those who abruptly stop taking antidepressants after using them for at least six weeks suffer from a variety of often flulike symptoms, including insomnia, lethargy, anxiety/hyperarousal, dysphoria, dizziness, gastrointestinal upset, and nausea. Symptoms typically start within three days of stopping the drugs, and patients who have taken the drugs for longer periods are more likely to suffer these problems. To be fair, symptoms are generally mild and usually stop after a couple of weeks, but they have been commonly associated with missed time at work and, occasionally, hospitalization.[135] It all makes sense—stopping the drugs quickly leads to a dramatic decline in the amount of serotonin in the synapses, which affects other areas in which serotonin is involved, such as diet, sleep, emotions, aggression, and sensory perceptions. "I feel like my brain is floating in Jell-O, slamming into the sides of my skull every time I move my head or eyes," one such sufferer wrote on an Internet Web site dedicated to antidepressant withdrawal problems. Some patients describe the feeling of shock through their arms and legs, as if they'd been zapped by electricity, called "lightning-bolt syndrome." "The feeling can be really abrupt, like a quick jerk of the muscle," says Richard Shelton, a psychiatrist at Vanderbilt University. "It's not painful, but it can be very frightening to people."[136] Paxil and Effexor, which have shorter half-lives than most antidepressants (meaning that the drug is flushed out of the body more quickly), have higher rates of antidepressant discontinuation syndrome than Prozac, which has a very long half-life. Off-label uses of the drugs for conditions unrelated to mental illness—such as irritable bowel syndrome, weight loss, headaches, insomnia—may be associated with a higher risk of antidepressant discontinuation syndrome.[137] It would seem that the more dubious the reason for taking the medication, the more problematic the outcome and effect it has on the body.

The following is a story from a research psychologist from Oregon, describing his experience taking, and then trying to get off, antidepressants and other psychiatric drugs.

> I started taking antidepressants at age 19 when my mother sent me to see a psychiatrist because I was floundering in college. I realize now that I gave these well-intentioned doctors far too much credit and didn't question the strictly biological approach to treating my depression until the drugs started to poop out and I noticed that I was emotionally numb, overweight, sexless *and* depressed. I soldiered on, but then one day they stopped working in a rather dramatic fashion, and I ended up in a much, much worse state than my baseline depression. For eighteen months my doctor and I toyed with heroic polypharmacy until finally I was propped up enough to start graduate work in clinical psychology. I did wonderfully the first year academically. I was socially engaged and was running 25 miles a week but I didn't feel like me anymore. There was a palpable disconnect as well as many side effects that were concerning.
>
> Then I started to develop repeated hellish episodes of a potentially fatal condition called serotonin syndrome that included symptoms such as extreme muscle stiffness, mental confusion, and rage. Because of the long-standing side effects and the emergence of the serotonin syndrome, I began a long, slow, and painful taper off a cocktail of medication, which took nearly five years. During this time and through the present, I have experienced severe withdrawal symptoms including mood swings, twitching, jerking, stiffness, vomiting for six weeks,

> insomnia, significant cognitive deficits, profound fatigue, motivation problems, and a cartoonish inability to manage stress. Needless to say I had never experienced *any* of these symptoms before starting to taper off this God-awful dope. Over the two years I've been drug free, I have experienced improvement, but my functioning really hasn't changed. There is reason to believe that I will continue to improve over the next year, but my future is a huge blinking question mark.

Another devastating side effect has been found to be far more common than once thought. It is well known among clinicians that in people who suffer from bipolar disorder, antidepressants can trigger a manic state, or "mixed state" that oscillates between mania and depression.. Clinicians need to exercise particular vigilance with bipolar patients who are taking SSRIs, often needing to ensure that they take an additional mood-stabilizing medication. Typical signs of mania include not sleeping for days on end, "pressured speech" (talking so rapidly that all the words rush together), using street drugs, bursts of activity and "creativity" like painting or writing all night (although usually patients are so sloppily deranged that nothing comes out of these efforts), and compromised judgment about money and sex. Antidepressants can induce such states in people who are already highly vulnerable to them. A group of Yale psychiatrists reviewed the charts of all consecutive admissions—more than five hundred patients altogether—to the inpatient psychiatric unit of Yale–New Haven Hospital. Eight percent of the patients admitted to the inpatient unit fit the profile of antidepressant-induced mania or psychosis. Their results were consistent with an earlier study showing that 11 percent of patients on the unit were hospitalized because of antidepressant-related psychosis and mania.[138] These are remarkably high figures that, in my experience, would surprise even most clinicians familiar with the risk of SSRIs for bipolar patients.

Perhaps the most disturbing SSRI side effect comes to those who do not even ingest them. A 2006 study showed that about 30 percent of infants exposed to SSRIs before birth experience some symptoms of withdrawal from the drugs. In 13 percent of the babies, those symptoms were severe. Problems included tremor, gastrointestinal upset, sleep disturbance, high-pitched crying, accelerated breathing, and temperature instability.[139]

And of course nobody really knows the long-term side effects of SSRIs—that is, the impact of taking them for decades and decades. It is simply uncharted territory. Even Peter Kramer acknowledged this in a far more subdued interview a few years ago: "My worry is the lack of testing of long-term usage . . . When a medicine goes from being used by a few people to being used by hundreds of millions of people, for long periods of time, there have to be studies that look at the public health implications and the effects of long-term use . . . It's true that we don't really know the long-term effects on the brain."[140] And SSRIs, of course, run through the whole body, not just the brain. Ninety-five percent of the serotonin in the body actually resides in the intestines, where it acts as a signaling mechanism to the brain.[141] The heart, too, has serotonin receptors. No one knows what impact decades of SSRI use might have on those organs.

Perhaps most significantly, and forebodingly, in the late 1990s, David Healy put Kramer's "cosmetic pharmacology" claims to the test. He recruited students who had no history of mental illness whatsoever for a study at his university in Wales and gave them antidepressants. Ten percent of what was an admittedly small sample developed horribly disturbing suicidal and homicidal tendencies, completely alien to anything they had ever experienced. One person imagined slitting her throat and bleeding to death in bed next to her partner. Another person decided to throw herself in front of a car, and it was only because of a chance phone call that she was stopped.[142] While still retaining belief in their clinical efficacy when used with caution and oversight, Healy has since become one of the SSRI industry's biggest attackers.

The commerce of mood certainly can make a lot of people wealthy, but apparently it doesn't solve all ills.

In 2003, the chief executive officer of Pfizer, Henry "Hank" McKinnell, sat in his corner office in midtown Manhattan. McKinnell was paid $9.7 million a year in earnings[143] and ultimately received $200 million in retirement and deferred compensation.[144]

It was raining outside, and McKinnell was feeling blue. "We're the industry and the company that nobody loves," he said. "I'm just kind of puzzled at how we got here." Lamenting the fact that politicians increasingly like to blame Big Pharma for government deficits and that his company in particular is under scrutiny from shareholders, McKinnell said, "I call it generalized anxiety disorder," perhaps not fully realizing he was citing a diagnosis upon which Pfizer and other companies have made a tidy profit.[145]

CHAPTER THREE

The Triumph of Biological Psychiatry

The path that psychiatry has traversed in the past one hundred years has been extraordinary. Psychiatry has gone from "the concern of a small a group of alienists"[1] who treated only the most severely mentally ill deep inside asylum walls to dominating corporate profit margins and becoming a staple of the airwaves and middle-class conversations. Psychiatry, which for most of its existence nobody of sound mind wanted anything much to do with, now touches most people's lives, directly or indirectly. When Tom Cruise and Brooke Shields battle over the use of antidepressants for postpartum depression, it is national news.

The history of American psychiatry can be divided into three overlapping eras: a progression from Asylum Psychiatry, to Community Psychiatry, to Corporate Psychiatry.[2] Roughly speaking, Asylum Psychiatry can be said to have begun around 1800, with the founding of a series of hospitals for the mentally ill—Spring Grove State Hospital in Maryland in 1798, the Hartford Retreat in Connecticut in 1824, Manhattan State Hospital in New York City in 1825. Asylum Psychiatry grew tremendously over the course of the nineteenth century—by 1904, there were 150,000 patients in U.S. psychiatric hospitals—and reached its peak about 1950, with a census well over half a million.[3] The true beginning of Community Psychiatry ironically can be tied to the invention of Thorazine, the first antipsychotic medication, in the early 1950s, which, for better or worse, led to the opening of the doors of the mental hospitals. Long-term psychiatric patients were let free into the community. The initial tremors of Corporate Psychiatry were felt in the late 1960s and into the 1970s, when Valium became the top-selling drug in America, but this was just a flirtation compared to what was to come later. Corporate Psychiatry began in earnest in 1988 with the introduction of Prozac.

In its improbable odyssey from the back wards of asylums to the boardrooms of corporations, psychiatry has gone from being invisible to visible. The ability to *see psychiatry* at any level has proved pivotal and momentous. For its first century at least, psychiatry has been conducted in the shadows: engaged with murky mental processes; taking place in concealed, often exclusive offices; its confidentiality protected by law and professional ethics; its methods "intimate and private," and "resistant to exposure."[4] But now psychiatry is everywhere, on television, in the movies, on television ads, and most significantly, in our bloodstreams.

Asylum Psychiatry has historically been two things—one of them perfectly well-intentioned and generally benign, and the other horrific. The initial impetus of the asylum movement was to provide retreats, often in the solace of nature, where, in the absence of any actual evidence-based treatments, patients could at least be left alone in a tranquil setting. To the credit of some of the early crusaders, prime real estate in sylvan settings was allocated for the most vulnerable and impoverished citizens. The state psychiatric hospital in Connecticut, for example, is situated on rolling hills overlooking the Connecticut River, arguably the most beautiful property in the valley. On the other hand, there is an equally long tradition in the asylums of the provision of the most wretched treatments imaginable. In 1728, making an observation that has since been echoed repeatedly by just about every intelligent observer of psychiatric institutions, Daniel Defoe wrote that life in an asylum was enough to drive anyone crazy: "If they are not mad when they go to these cursed Houses, they are soon made so by barbarous usage they there suffer . . . Is it not enough to make anyone mad to be suddenly clap'd up, stripp'd, whipp'd, ill fed and worse . . . ?"[5]

In the 1948 book *The Shame of the States*, the pioneering investigative journalist Albert Deutsch wrote that state mental hospitals were like "Nazi concentration camps at Belsen and Buchenwald . . . buildings swarming with naked humans herded like cattle and treated with less concern, pervaded by a fetid odor so heavy, so nauseating, that the stench seemed to have almost a physical existence of its own." Not uncommonly, patients were sterilized so as to permanently halt the moral contagion of their illness. This was often done under the rule of law. In 1927, the Supreme Court, by an eight-to-one margin, approved the sterilization of moral defectives. Oliver Wendell Holmes wrote in his decision, "It is better for all the world, if instead of waiting to execute degenerate offspring for crime, or to let them starve for their imbecility, society can prevent those who are manifestly unfit from continuing their kind."[6] Editorials in *The New York Times* and *The New England Journal of Medicine* endorsed the practice. By 1945, 45,000 Americans had been sterilized, 21,000 of whom were psychiatric patients in state facilities.[7] Afterward, one patient wrote: "I shall ever bemoan the fact that I shall never have a son to bear my name, to take my place, and to be a prop in my old age."[8]

In 1916, Dr. Henry Cotton of Trenton State Hospital, believing that germs from tooth decay led to insanity, removed patients' teeth and other body parts, such as the bowels, which he thought might be the causes of their madness. In so doing, he killed almost half of his patients—more than one hundred people.[9] Cotton's practices were covered up by the hospital board and the leading figure in American psychiatry of the day, Adolf Meyer, and Cotton was also allowed to continue practicing at the hospital for almost another twenty years. At his eulogy in 1933, Meyer lauded Cotton's "extraordinary record of achievement."[10]

Harvard-trained doctors John Talbott and Kenneth Tillotson, somehow under the impression that psychosis could be expunged by extreme thermal measures, wrapped patients in freezing blankets so that their body temperatures fell ten to twenty degrees below normal. (Tillotson later gained notoriety for administering botched electroshock therapy to Sylvia Plath, who committed suicide shortly thereafter. He failed to provide anesthetic, resulting in the poet's being semielectrocuted.)[11] In 1933, the psychiatrist Manfred Sakel of Vienna famously induced hypoglycemia in patients via the injection of insulin, thereby putting his patients into an insulin coma. Insulin therapy, as it was known, was considered state-of-the art treatment and written up in textbooks. One commentator wrote in 1939: "every self-respecting go-ahead hospital had its insulin unit."[12]

Not to mention the lobotomy, which was invented by the Portuguese neurologist Egas Moniz on November 12, 1935, when he performed the first what he called a "leucotomy," or "white cut." Moniz had been turned down for one Nobel Prize and was interested in making a splash with a new and decisive treatment. After hearing a lecture that conjectured that the prefrontal cortex was the site of psychopathology, he decided to try out a method of destroying that part of the brain on his patients. A few years later, in 1939, while working in his office, Moniz was shot, quite appropriately it would seem, multiple times by a disgruntled former patient. Moniz was partially paralyzed for the remainder of his life. Nonetheless, for his efforts, Moniz did indeed win the Nobel Prize in Physiology or Medicine in 1949.[13]

The American champion of the lobotomy, Walter Freeman, roamed the country as a veritable Johnny Appleseed of the technique, to which he added his own refinements, which amounted to jamming an ice pick through the patient's eye sockets and destroying the frontal lobes. In 1951, Freeman visited psychiatric hospitals in seventeen states and conducted demonstrations of his work in Puerto Rico, Curaçao, and Canada. Freeman became able to perform a surgery in less than ten minutes and perfected the technique so that he could insert picks into both eyes at once.[14] A successful operation, in Freeman's view, was one in which the patient became adjusted at "the level of a domestic invalid or household pet."[15] Between 1935 and 1950, 20,000 American psychiatric patients were subjected to lobotomies, or, as it was more gently called, "psychosurgery." What led to the demise of the lobotomy era was not any newfound compassion or enlightenment, but simply the emergence of antipsychotic drugs that made psychosurgery "redundant."[16]

In the United States, Community Psychiatry began when the profession took its first tentative steps into office practice between the world wars. The emigration of European psychoanalysts after World War I, and particularly after World War II, led to the establishment of office-based practices, particularly in large eastern cities like New York, Boston, and Philadelphia. So influential and revered were these analysts that the influence and prestige of the field moved away from the academy and into office practice over the course of the 1950s and 1960s. By 1955, more than 80 percent of American psychiatrists worked in private practice.[17] Now the prestige of the field is squarely back in the academy, and more specifically, in the laboratory.

As with Asylum Psychiatry, there have been two prongs of American Community Psychiatry: one has proved a great success, and the other became a national disgrace. For the worried well, the 1960s through the 1990s saw an explosion of nonpsychiatrist therapists (social workers, clinical psychologists, addiction counselors) who treated an ever-expanding proportion of the population. By the early 1980s, about 10 percent of Americans were being treated for mental problems each year, adding up to more than 300 million office visits.[18] As noted, Community Psychiatry for the seriously mentally ill began with the introduction of Thorazine, which led in one to two decades to the mass depopulation of the asylums. At first this was thought to be a wonderful development. Biologically minded psychiatrists thought they were setting patients free by giving them a medication that finally appeared to work and then sending them on their way. For socially minded psychiatrists, letting the patients into the community was an act of liberation from the oppression of institution and the hierarchies of medical care. For their part, state governments were only too happy to divest themselves of the expense of running massive networks of long-term care facilities. For all the high expectations and lofty rhetoric, the reality was that the effectiveness of the drugs was overestimated and the necessity of appropriate community support for patients was underestimated or ignored. The goal of John F. Kennedy's Community Mental Health Act to create a national network of outpatient clinics proved too lofty. The clinics quickly became co-opted by therapy sessions for the middle-class worried well, not the seriously mentally ill, and funding eventually withered during the prosecution of the Vietnam War. Kennedy's death, too, certainly played a part. He was an early advocate of community treatment, influenced no doubt by the experience of his own sister, Rosemary, who was developmentally disabled and mentally ill, and who herself had undergone a lobotomy. Eventually, there was simply no place for patients to go but the parks, the bus stations, the public libraries, the emergency rooms, and the homeless shelters. Deinstitutionalization coincided with the arrival of AIDS and the emergence of "crack" cocaine in the early 1980s, and the numbers of the homeless mentally ill rose dramatically across the country.

Both Asylum Psychiatry and Community Psychiatry have been swept away by a new Corporate Psychiatry. Aslyums, today called state hospitals, now house about 5 percent of the patients they did at their peak; Community Psychiatry is being eroded by managed care and the national obsession with psychiatric medications. Corporate Psychiatry, with its blockbuster products and its high-tech glow, is where the juice is now.

How did psychiatry undergo such a remarkable transformation? How did it go from nothing—or, rather, worse than nothing: unspeakable treatment in asylums—to *Oprah*, morning talk shows, and Wall Street?

Many factors of course have contributed, but the key to all of them has been the direct effect of the filtering into public consciousness, in simplistic and often misunderstood form, of the effects of a revolution that has taken place in academic psychiatry in the last twenty years—the ascendancy and now complete dominance of biological psychiatry, or neuropsychiatry, in universities across the country. All of this has contributed to a new public image of psychiatry as a real branch of medicine and a bona fide science built on white-coated certitude. Finally, psychiatry is Big Science. It is the suspicion, now apparently confirmed in the view of the public, that all our behavior finally comes down to molecules and transmission between those molecules and that psychiatry in some profound way is starting to unlock those mysteries. It is the all too hasty belief that biological psychiatry has emerged into something akin to physics and chemistry, reassuring in its rules and clarity. As Paul Rabinow, a Berkeley anthropologist put it, "More and more stories about who we are and how we live are becoming molecular."[19]

Steven Rose, a British neurobiologist, says, "The power of molecular talk [in biology, neuroscience, and psychiatry] is very seductive because it seems somehow much closer to the hard sciences."[20] Rose goes on to point out that physics is always the measuring stick. In the development of western science, physics and chemistry came first, and thereby framed what we believe a science should be. Biology came later and aspired to fit these earlier paradigms. This is all well and good, but the difficulty lies in the fact that biology is inherently messy—and neurobiology messier still. The completion of the Human Genome Project in 2001, also, by association, has served to bolster psychiatry's newfound scientific image. That a rough draft of the human genetic makeup has been developed contributes to a popular belief that psychiatric disorders proceed in neat Mendelian inheritable patterns. But if anything has been gleaned for the last two decades of work in the genetics of psychiatric disorders, it is that it is a terribly complex business. No single gene for psychiatric disorders have been found and likely will never be found. Psychiatric disorders are almost certainly the dialectical product of an infinitely complex dialogue between genes and the environment.

Another contributor to the bolstered profile of psychiatry is the relatively recent emergence of randomized clinical trials (RCTs), which have become the ne plus ultra of psychiatry and all of medicine. It was only in 1948 that the first double-blind randomized trial was reported, meaning that neither the subjects nor the researchers know who belongs to the control group or the experimental group. (It happened to be for the use of a drug for treating tuberculosis.)[21] While RCTs are a dramatic improvement, they are far from being worthy of our absolute faith. When the first two thousand RCTs for the treatment of schizophrenia were reviewed, it was discovered that most trials were significantly flawed by a number of problems, such as inadequate sample size, too short a duration, inconsistent evaluation methods, and poor reporting of data. Only 1 percent of the trials were given top marks on a one-to-five scale of quality.[22] Not to mention the fact that about one-third of biomedical scientists have admitted to questionable research practices, such as changing experimental methods and reporting based on the preferences of their funders.[23]

There is also a subtle inherent logical limitation in RCTs. RCTs are not set up to confirm how exactly a medication or treatment is effective, but rather to confirm the null hypothesis—that is, that the intervention or medication is no better than nothing at all. In the standard RCT, one compares a treatment arm with a control arm, in which no treatment is provided. When a particular agent in an RCT is successful, all that has been demonstrated is that the treatment was in some way better than no treatment at all. In other words, unless it is independently evident that the treatment addresses the illness—in the way, for example, that penicillin treats pneumonia—then one does not actually learn much from the trial.[24] One has merely found evidence of an association between events but not an explanation as to how those events linked.

As a result of psychiatry's long-anticipated entry into the realm of Big Science, earlier paradigms in academic psychology and psychiatry, mushy-headed things like old-fashioned psychoanalysis and behaviorism and psychotherapeutic techniques have been jettisoned—tragically too soon, it turns out—like so many rotting vegetables.

It is startling how rapidly the shift occurred. Until 1950, the predominant theories about how the brain functioned were electrical, not chemical.[25] When the first psychiatric drugs were discovered, no one had a clue what a neurotransmitter was. It was only in 1965 that the first biological theory of a major psychiatric disorder was published.[26] Only forty years ago, psychiatric disorders were overwhelmingly considered a product of bad mothering, poor adjustment, repressed sexuality, and poor attachments to others. Not genes and chemicals, but nurture and environmental explanations of mental predicaments ruled the day. And until quite recently, biological psychiatry was often seen as totalitarian and ruthless in its oppressive force. If one didn't comply with the rules of society or rules of the wards, one was shocked into compliance—or, at the very least emasculated. (Think *A Clockwork Orange* and *One Flew Over the Cuckoo's Nest.*)

In 1968, the offices of Jean Delay, one of the most eminent figures in the history of psychopharmacology (indeed, he invented the term) were ransacked by students at the University of Paris. The students considered Delay, who had presided over the early testing of Thorazine, to be a creator of *camisoles chimiques*—"chemical straitjackets." When the university responded to demands by the students, Delay resigned in protest. In 1969, students occupied the psychiatry department at Tokyo University and forced a prominent psychiatrist in Japan from office for biological research he had done in the 1950s. Ultimately, they halted all research for a decade. In 1971, at McGill University in Canada, Heinz Lehman, the first champion of Thorazine in North America, had a cream pie thrown in his face by his opponent in a debate on the biological treatments of mental illness. Lehman kept on speaking.[27]

As Tom Wolfe put it, those echoes you heard in the middle of the night in the late 1980s and early 1990s were the sounds of departments of psychiatry and psychology in universities all across the country taking down their placards and putting up new ones, saying Departments of *Neuro*psychology and *Neuro*psychiatry."[28] Simultaneously, new shiny buildings for neuroscience programs were built, now numbering in the hundreds across the country: Harvard's Interfaculty Initiative on Mind, Brain and Behavior; Columbia's Center for Neurobiology and Behavior; Princeton's Center for the Study of Brain, Mind and Behavior; Dartmouth's Center for Cognitive Neuroscience. Neuroscience is now arguably the hottest field in academia. The number of new PhDs more than doubled between the 1980s and 1990s.[29] When Leon Eisenberg, now an eminence in psychiatry, joined the Society for Neuroscience in 1971, he became its ninety-first member.[30] In 2006, there were 37,000 members in the society, with almost 40 percent under the age of thirty-five.[31] By contrast, the American Psychoanalytic Association holds steady at about 3,500 members. The Society for Neuroscience also reports the astonishing fact that in 2004 there were 6.7 million downloads of the articles in its journal, *The Journal of Neuroscience*—up 2.4 million from the previous year![32] It is unlikely that there is another academic journal in the world that could claim such numbers. To keep up with the huge popular demand for neuroscientific information, *Scientific American* launched a new magazine, *Scientific American Mind*, in 2004.

The torrent of money flowing into the neuro world can only be described in a series of superlatives. Columbia recently announced plans for the Jerome L. Greene Science Center, a neuroscience research center, made possible with a $200 million bequest, which was the largest private gift received by any American university for the creation of a single facility. In 2000, MIT received a commitment of $350 million for the McGovern Institute for Brain Research, one of the largest gifts ever given to a university. MIT followed that up with the announcement of another $50 million bequest for brain studies, the largest bequest ever given to that institution by a private foundation. The McKnight Foundation, supported with money from the 3M Company, has funded brain research centers at the universities of Florida, Miami, and Alabama, as well as scholars at universities all over the country. Neuroscience is one of the principal areas of focus of the Howard Hughes Medical Institute, the endowment of which is $16 billion (derived from the 1985 sale of Hughes Aircraft to General Motors). The emphasis on neuroscience is appropriate, as the institute's founder, the aviator, industrialist, film tycoon, and iconoclast Howard Hughes, famously and prodigiously suffered from obsessive-compulsive disorder. Government funding has followed suit. Funding for the National Institute of Mental Health, $90 million in 1976, reached $1.4 billion in 2006.[33] And just between 1998 and 2003, that budget doubled.[34]

Given the special prestige that neuroscience and biological psychiatry presently occupy in our culture, it is hard to fathom that psychoanalysis enjoyed that exact same level of prestige and influence less than fifty years ago. It is now largely a cultural afterthought except among those remaining people who subscribe to what has been called the "Woody Allen syndrome": wealthy people on the Upper West and East Sides of Manhattan and a few other similarly well-heeled urban areas around the country. Writing in 1959, the heyday of psychoanalysis in America, the sociologist Philip Rieff observed: "In America today, Freud's intellectual influence is greater than that of any other thinker. He presides over the mass media, the college classroom, the chatter at parties, the playgrounds of the middle classes."[35] The literary critic Lionel Trilling, in 1947, called Freud's legacy "the only systematic account of the human mind, which, in point of subtlety and complexity, of interest and tragic power, deserves to stand beside the chaotic mass of psychological insights that literature has accumulated through the centuries."[36]

Freud of course reigned over American psychiatry in the 1950s and 1960s. In that era, it was virtually impossible for the head of any respectable department of psychiatry not to be a psychoanalyst, just as today it's a virtual impossibility for one not to be a neuroscientist. When Leon Eisenberg dared utter a few words challenging the scientific basis of psychoanalysis at a conference in 1962, "there was a veritable stampede of department chairmen to the floor microphones . . . Just about every eminent figure present rose to defend the primacy of psychoanalysis as the 'the basic science' of psychiatry."[37] As a trainee in the early 1960s, a young psychiatrist was warned by his supervisors about giving medication to people with catatonic schizophrenia "because it would muck up transference," a reference to the process by which the patient projects feelings and emotions onto the therapist.[38] These days he'd likely be told not to do therapy at all.

While psychoanalysis was introduced to the United States in 1909 when Freud (accompanied by Carl Jung) delivered a famous lecture at Clark University, its influence grew fairly slowly for the next three decades. The "shell shock" of the survivors of World War I led to some novel treatments (some innovative and compassionate, others as horrific as the war itself), as well as the rise of the "mental hygiene" movement of the 1920s and 1930s; the experience of Vietnam veterans led directly to the entry of posttraumatic stress disorder into the revised psychiatric diagnostic manual in 1980; and a considerable amount of the news coverage of the Iraq War has addressed the (deteriorating) mental status of the troops, with calls for more assessment, treatment, and general vigilance for their fragile psyches.*

World War II was the first conflict in which psychiatry played a major role. For the first time, all American soldiers were screened by psychiatrists and physicians for their mental fitness for war. The screening tool was partially developed by Harry Stack Sullivan, a legendary psychoanalyst.[40] An astounding number of men—at least 1.1 million and perhaps as many as 1.9 million—were rejected because of psychiatric and neurological problems, which amounts to 12 percent of the 15 million men evaluated. In practice, most of the screenings lasted less than two minutes and were administered by physicians with no psychiatric training.[41] The war, of course, also produced an unprecedented stream of new patients for psychiatry: an endless supply of, to use the euphemism of the day, "battle fatigued" soldiers suffering from guilt, anxiety, and terrifying flashbacks. There were a remarkable 1.1 million admissions for psychiatric disorders in military hospitals over the course of the war.[42] (How deeply hidden this part of the war experience has been kept is a profound reflection of the stigma attached to mental suffering at that time.) To treat this unprecedented anguish, there existed no coherent system of care other than psychoanalysis. Also, psy-

*See Pat Barker's World War I novel, *Regeneration*, based on historical figures, for a wonderful exploration of the treatments—both horrific and palliative—of shell shock. The term *shell shock*, incidentally, derives from the theory of the day that the impact of the shells led to tears in the spinal cord, which in turn led to the nervous problems of traumatized soldiers. The competing psychoanalytic explanation was that the conditions of war caused soldiers to regress to an infantile condition, whereby commanding officers became father or older brother figures "in a manner that aroused primal sadistic and homosexual impulses."[39]

choanalysis, with its emphasis on internal conflict, memories, dreams, and nightmares seemed suitably oriented to address the symptoms of "battle fatigue."[43]

Psychoanalytic practices and concepts were directly infused into military policy in 1943 when William Menninger, an outspoken and articulate member of the Topeka Psychoanalytic Society, was appointed chief military psychiatrist. In two short years, Menninger assertively brought psychiatry into the mainstream of military life. Menninger's ability to act as psychiatry's salesman, both during and after the war, was helped immeasurably by his hypernormal, squeaky-clean Chamber of Commerce image. As *Time* wrote in 1948, "Dr. Will Menninger himself is a convincing explanation of why the public is getting less skittish about psychiatry. Plainly neither a crackpot nor a foreigner, Psychiatrist Menninger is a big (6 ft. 1 in., 189 lbs.), friendly 'nice guy' . . . There is not a touch of the Hollywood-style, burning-eyed psychiatrist about Dr. Will . . ."[44] In 1944, Menninger issued a bulletin for army physicians, "Neuropsychiatry for the General Medical Officer," in which the role of the subconscious in symptoms was explained, as well as the influence of infancy and childhood on adult character. Menninger's recommended treatment methods for war neurosis included hypnosis and psychoanalytic therapy.

In 1945, Menninger introduced an entirely new diagnostic nomenclature for the field. He created new categories specifically geared to incorporate the war experience—such as "transient personality reactions to acute and special stress," which included "combat exhaustion" and "acute situational maladjustment" as diagnoses. The section on neurosis was lifted directly from Freud, with sections on repression, conversion (the expression of psychological distress into physical complaints), and displacement (the shifting of emotions from the original object to a more acceptable substitute). Menninger's taxonomy had far-reaching influence beyond the war, becoming the basis for the American Psychiatric Association's first diagnostic manual in 1952, the direct predecessor of today's *Diagnostic and Statistical Manual of Mental Disorders*, the best-selling "bibles" of contemporary psychiatry. Not everybody appreciated the new influence of psychiatry in the military.

Concerned about maintaining adequate troop levels on the front, General George Marshall complained that while a psychiatrist would consider a soldier suffering from battle fatigue as a "hospital patient," to the line officer he was a malingerer. Marshall objected to the "hyper-considerate professional attitude" of the psychiatrist.[45]

The war also saw the advent of new treatment techniques. Group therapy was invented by beleaguered and overwhelmed medical staff and showed great promise for soldiers suffering from what we would now call posttraumatic stress disorder. It is has been suggested that one of the reasons that group therapy worked so well, particularly for British troops, is the manner in which it broke down the hierarchies of military life and the prewar social structure.[46] Medical staff rarely wore white coats; patients and staff referred to each other by their first names. The experience and trauma of war bolstered belief in the environmental causations of mental illness. Meanwhile, genetic and hereditary explanations lost substantial ground in the face of the tragic evidence of the damage that experience could do.[47]

In the optimistic glow immediately following the war, Americans really did believe that psychoanalysis could help make the postwar world a better place. In 1945, Menninger could write that "psychiatry, for better or worse, is receiving a tremendously increased interest. This is manifest on all sides by articles in magazines, in the newspapers, frequent references to psychiatry and psychiatric problems on the radio and in the movies."[48] Demand for psychiatric treatment grew tremendously. For the first time, the image of the mysterious but all-knowing analyst became a stock-in-trade of cartoonists.[49] There was much eloquent writing by analysts and their followers about the transformative possibilities of therapy. A small group of psychiatrists and impassioned laypersons lobbied for and helped secure the passage of the Mental Health Act of 1946, which led to the establishment of the National Institute of Mental Health. Hence, *Life* magazine wrote in 1947:

> A boom has overtaken the once obscure and much maligned profession of psychoanalysis. It is part of the larger boom which simultaneously has engulfed the whole science of psychiatry . . .

> and which has made the 4,011 accredited psychiatrists about the most sought-after members of the entire medical profession . . . And of all psychiatrists, the comparative handful of analysts . . . seem to be the most heavily besieged . . . [T]his . . . reflects in the increase in popular knowledge and acceptance of psychiatry, and especially psychoanalysis, as a cure.[50]

Over the course of the 1950s the terms *psychiatrist* and *psychoanalyst* became synonymous in the American popular imagination. In fact, there was only a tiny cadre of psychoanalysts—there were no more than 1,400 practicing analysts *in the world* in 1957[51]—at the core of this movement, but their numbers were enhanced by the addition of a throng of psychologists and social workers, who, while technically not analysts, brought psychoanalytic approaches to their work. The newly fashionable image of the analyst was reflected in the popular cinema. The kindly and wise doctor prevailed. In 1957's *The Three Faces of Eve*, Joanne Woodward's multiple-personality disorder was cured by therapy with a psychiatrist played by Lee J. Cobb. John Huston directed the hagiographic *Freud* in 1962 (starring Montgomery Clift as the great man), and a year later, Gregory Peck starred in *Captain Newman, MD*, a portrait of a gifted and wise analyst, based on the true history of Ralph Greenson, the Los Angeles psychiatrist who treated Marilyn Monroe. Such enthusiastic portrayals were no doubt a reflection of the fact that the number of Hollywood actors, directors, and producers being treated by psychoanalysis were "legion."[52] When Karl Menninger, William's brother, visited Los Angeles in 1953, he was feted by twenty movie stars who had been treated at the Menninger Foundation.[53]

In 1961, *The Atlantic* devoted an entire issue to psychiatry in American life. The introduction stated: "The impact of the [psychoanalytic] revolution has been incalculable. To an extent not paralleled elsewhere, psychoanalysis and psychiatry in general have influenced medicine, the arts and criticism, popular entertainment, advertising, the rearing of children, sociology, anthropology, legal thought and practice, manners and mores, even organized religion."[54] Shortly thereafter, the central dilemma of the psychoanalyst was identified in the journal *Daedalus:*

there weren't enough of them to be everywhere at once. As T. M. Luhrmann wrote of that era, "The assumption seemed to be that if a psychiatrist *could* be everywhere, he *would* be able to solve all social ills."[55] There were serious discussions that if only statesmen were analyzed, there would be no more wars, and articles appeared in psychiatric journals about the psychoanalytic implications of Kennedy's death for the nation.[56]

How soon, and how easily, it would all crumble away.

It is fashionable now in academic psychiatry to condemn the fancies of the last century. "All sciences have to pass through an ordeal by quackery," wrote the psychologist Hans Eysenck. "Chemistry had to slough off the fetters of alchemy. The brain sciences had to disengage themselves from the tenets of phrenology . . . Psychology and psychiatry too will have to abandon the pseudo-science of psychoanalysis . . . and undertake the arduous task of transforming their disciplines into a genuine science."[57] "Psychology itself is dead," writes Michael Gazzaniga, director of the Center for Cognitive Neuroscience at Dartmouth, in *The Mind's Past.* "Today the mind sciences are the province of evolutionary biologists, cognitive scientists, neuroscientists, psychophysicists, computer scientists—you name it . . . The odd thing is that everyone but its practitioners know about the death of psychology."[58] Freud, incidentally, predicted this. That is, he predicted his own death. In 1924's *Beyond the Pleasure Principle*, he wrote about psychoanalysis: "The deficiencies in our description would probably vanish if we were already in a position to replace the psychological terms with physiological or chemical ones. We may expect [physiology and chemistry] to give the most surprising information, and we cannot guess what answers it will return in a few dozen years of questions we have put to it. They may be of a kind that will blow away the whole of our artificial structure of hypothesis."[59]

Two developments sum up the revolution—the discovery of drugs that actually work, at least for some people, and brain imaging.

Thorazine was the first drug to work. Its invention has been called one of the seminal events in human history and the beginning of the revolution in psychiatry, comparable to the introduction of penicillin in general medicine.[60] It was of course discovered by accident, and when it worked, no one had any idea why. In 1952, Henri Laborit, a French surgeon, was looking for a way to reduce surgical shock in patients. Much of the shock came from anesthesia; Laborit reasoned that if he could use less anesthetic, patients could recover more quickly. Casting about for a solution, Laborit tried Thorazine, a shelved medication that had been developed a number of years before to fight allergies. Laborit noticed an immediate change in his patients' mental states. They became relaxed and seemingly indifferent to the surgery awaiting them. Laborit thought Thorazine might be helpful to psychiatric patients, but at that time, "no one in their right mind in psychiatry was working with drugs. You used shock or various psychotherapies," according to psychiatrist Heinz Lehman,[61] Thorazine's first champion in North America (and in whose face the pie was thrown at the debate at McGill University).

Laborit told his brother-in-law, Pierre Deniker, a psychiatrist, about Thorazine, and Deniker tried it on his most agitated, uncontrollable patients on the back wards of a Parisian psychiatric hospital. This was a startlingly novel idea. "Those cases were in the back wards and that was it. The notion you could ever do anything about [them] had never occurred to anyone," said John Young,[62] an executive at the American drug company that bought the rights to Thorazine a couple of years later, only to first put it on the market as an antivomiting treatment.[63] Deniker's colleague Jean Perrin gave Thorazine to a barber from Lyon who had been hospitalized for years and been unresponsive to any intervention. When given Thorazine, the barber awoke from his stuporous state and told his doctor that he now knew who and where he was and he wanted to go home and get back to work. Perrin hid his shock and asked the patient to give him a shave, which the patient did, perfectly. Another patient, suffering from catatonic schizophrenia, had been frozen in various postures for years. He responded to the drug in one day. Within twenty-four hours, he greeted the staff by name and asked for billiard balls to juggle. Many of the hopeless cases who took

Thorazine were transformed to previously inconceivable levels of calm and reasonableness, and some were released entirely. The change was apparent even to people living near the hospital, who noticed a huge drop in noise coming from the institution.[64]

After Deniker and others got over their initial shock and enthusiasm, it became clear over time what antipsychotics can do—and what they can't. In no fashion do they cure the illness, but for many, if not most, people with psychotic disorders like schizophrenia, they do help to make the condition eminently more tolerable. In many cases, the medications, quite literally, lower the volume. Many patients have told me that the drugs dampen the sounds of the voices that plague them, reducing the screams and rants to faint echoes and occasionally drowning them out entirely. Psychiatrists compare the way in which psychiatric drugs help, when they are effective, to how insulin works for people with diabetes: although far from a cure, they do help the majority of patients manage, and allow them, for the most part, to function, or function better. Or, as *Scientific American* more clinically put it: "Antipsychotics stop all symptoms in only about 20% of patients. Two thirds gain some relief yet remain symptomatic throughout life, and the remainder shows no significant response."[65] What also became evident over time were the incredibly harsh side effects of the first antipsychotics: involuntary muscle movements, endless pacing (or the "Thorazine shuffle," as it became known), and for some, a horrible restlessness, the feeling of needing to crawl out of one's skin.

Thorazine was brought to America by the drug company Smith Kline & French, and it was promptly given to almost all patients in all mental hospitals in the United States.[66] A colleague of mine was an orderly at Manhattan State Psychiatric Hospital when Thorazine was introduced. Every patient was put on the same dosage. He said the place was transformed in a day or two from bedlam to relative calm. From 1954, when Thorazine was approved by the FDA, through 1964, 50 million people took the drug—and Smith Kline's revenues doubled three times in over fifteen years.[67]

But with Thorazine and its many successors (it was but the first of a series of antipsychotic medications), American public mental hospitals by 1988 lost 80 percent of their patients from their historic height of more than half a million people in 1955.[68] With the arrival of Thorazine, psychoanalysis began to decline. A relative of Ludwig Binswanger, Freud's Swiss disciple and the director of a famous analytic clinic, was treated with medications by a young pharmacologically oriented German psychiatrist named Fritz Flügel. At the end of a very successful treatment, Binswanger told Flügel, "Fritz, with two pills, you destroyed a psychodynamic castle that took me fifty years to build." Binswanger's clinic closed in 1980.[69]

If Thorazine started the revolution, brain images finished it. While brain imaging has its origins with computerized tomography in the 1960s, its most spectacular contributions have occurred in the last fifteen years. Even when CT scans did reveal startling images in the 1970s—as did a landmark 1976 study that showed that the brains of people with schizophrenia had much larger ventricles than did "normals"—the results were received with doubt, as schizophrenia was assumed to be a psychological disease.[70] As George H. W. Bush's 1990 presidential proclamation announcing "The Decade of the Brain" put it, three things happened simultaneously in the 1980s that set up the miraculous pictures to come: technologies like PET (Positron Emission Tomography) scans and MRI (Magnetic Resonance Imaging) allowed researchers, for the first time, to observe the living brain; computer technology reached a level of sophistication sufficient to handle neuroscience data in a manner that reflected actual brain function; and discoveries at the molecular and cellular level of the brain shed greater light on how neurophysiological events translate into behavior, thought, and emotion. The first brain-imaging technologies, CT scans and MRI, were able to image brain *structure:* what the brain would look like if you could take it out from the skull and place it on a table.[71] MRI had the advantage of better-quality images, and there is no need to use ionizing radiation in the brain to create the images. The resolution of MRI is superb—it yields "slices" of brain that look as if they were obtained in a postmortem pathology lab. PET and SPECT (Single

Photon Emission Computed Tomography) scans, which came later, provide an image of brain activity, or *function*, by measuring blood flow in the brain as an index of brain activity. PET actually shows how neuroreceptors live in the brain, allowing one to see the distribution and number of receptors in particular areas of the brain, the concentration of neurotransmitters at the synapse, and the affinity of a receptor for a particular drug. PET specifically measures glucose metabolism, an indicator of which parts of the brain are using the most energy, which allows neuroscientists to undertake the process of mapping the neural basis of thought and emotion in the living brain.

But the most spectacular technology of all, fMRI—or Functional Magnetic Resonance Imaging—burst on the scene in the early 1990s. fMRI is unique in that it is able to provide images of both *structure and function*. It produces not just slices of the brain, but what are in effect extremely high-resolution movies of what the brain looks like when it is working. By measuring the proportion of oxygen in the blood, which is an indicator of brain activity, fMRI reveals which parts of the brain are being used most actively during a given task. These methods permit the observation of the brain as it is actually functioning as a mind: thinking, remembering, seeing, hearing, imagining, and experiencing pleasure or pain. Unlike earlier technologies, the total scan time is very short (one to two minutes), entirely noninvasive, and extraordinarily comprehensive: fMRI can measure brain responses at 100,000 locations. With the wonders of brain imaging, and in particular fMRI, the leading neuropsychologist Steven Pinker has written exuberantly, "Every facet of mind, from mental images to the moral sense, from mundane memories to acts of genius, has been tied to tracts of neural real estate . . . Using fMRI, scientists can tell whether the owner of a brain is imagining a face or a place. They can knock out a gene and prevent a mouse from learning, or insert extra copies and make it learn better."[72]

While the sudden visibility of the brain—the taking off of the shroud—has indeed been remarkable, the greater significance is perhaps more symbolic. Brain images are still far cruder than one would think after reading the sensational insights attributed to them in the science pages of newspapers and magazines. Neural events occur at a micrometer scale; whereas the images of fMRI, for example, are on the millimeter scale. That's sort of like watching a football game on a small television fifty yards away with your glasses off, and trying to identify the left tackle.

Second, it must be remembered that these are *secondary* images of blood flow and glucose in the brain and not of brain tissue itself. We seem to forget that it's not as if a camera is entering the brain and taking pictures of what's going on. At this point, the most that can be said is that brain imaging indirectly and very broadly measures the activity of groups of thousands of neurons when the brain is engaged in a physical or mental task. While there are some correlations between brain activity in certain regions and external, observable behavior, it is very hard to gauge what the pictures really mean. How does the flow of blood in parts of the brain correspond to feelings, moods, opinions, emotions, imagination? It remains a daunting task to create theories to "operationalize" what is going on underneath all the pretty pictures. The largest question of all, consciousness (which is, after all, the essence of being human), is completely untraveled territory. Whoever develops a true theory of consciousness will be the next Einstein, the next Freud, the next Copernicus.

The state of the art right now is that we can read brains—to some very crude extent—but we can't even begin to read minds. *The New York Times* asks, "Can Brain Scans See Depression?" and the answer is an overwhelming no. *The Wall Street Journal* science writer Sharon Begley has coined the term *cognitive paparazzi* to capture the hype and lack of substance that surrounds brain imaging.[73] "What does neuroscience know about how the brain makes decisions? Basically nothing," says Michael Gazzaniga. Another problem, Gazzaniga says, is that many brain imaging studies are based on averages of the scans of many patients. "The problem is if you go back to the individual scans, you will see wide variation in the part of the brain that's activated."[74] And if you were to do the same scans of the same activity a year later, you might get quite different results. (To be fair, however, concerns about retest reliability are much lower today than they were even a few years ago.)

"[The] community of scientists was excessively optimistic about how quickly imaging would have an impact on psychiatry," says Dr. Steven Hyman, a professor of neurobiology and provost at Harvard, as well as former director of the National Institute of Mental Health. "In their enthusiasm, people forgot that the human brain is the most complex object in the history of human inquiry, and it's not at all easy to see what's going wrong." There are currently no standard ways of treating or assessing mental illness based on brain images. Currently, the only unequivocal clinical use of imaging is raw abnormalities. "[The] only thing imaging can tell you is whether you have a brain tumor" or some other gross neurological damage, said Paul Root Wolpe of the University of Pennsylvania's Center for Bioethics.[75] The unfortunate fact remains that the most accurate way of gauging the thoughts and feelings of others is simply by asking people what they are thinking and feeling.

The fact that we can see anything in the brain has been revolutionary and explosive in its implications, but now that the public thinks we can see neurons, seemingly overnight, every aspect of human behavior, from the most trivial to the most profound, has acquired a neurological basis. It's a new neuro world we're living in. It helps no end that the term *neuro* seems to be able to attach itself to just about everything: neurobiology, neuropsychology, neuropsychiatry, neurophilosophy, neuroeconomics, neuromarketing, neuroethics, neurodiversity. Neurodiversity? Indeed. According to *The New York Times:* "As psychiatrists and neurologists uncover an ever-wider variety of brain wiring," a new kind of disability movement, calling for an acceptance of neurodiversity, has been born. Proponents of neurodiversity argue that "brain differences, like body differences, should be embraced," and appeal for a neurologically tolerant society.[76]

Neuropolitics? In the run-up to the 2004 presidential election, brain researchers showed Democrat and Republican voters a political ad while they were lying in an MRI machine. The researchers didn't bother to ask the voters what they thought of the ad—in this case a George W. Bush campaign spot that used 9/11 imagery. Instead, they observed which parts of the voters' brains were active as they watched. Democrats responded to the 9/11 imagery with far more activity in the amygdala—the part of the brain that responds to threats and danger—than did the Republicans. The UCLA neuroscientist who conducted the scans didn't think much of the traditional methodologies used by political scientists and consultants, like focus groups, to gauge the mood of the electorate. "It seemed so last century," Professor Joshua Freedman said. "Consultants were quoting Freud as if it was cutting edge. It was all about interpretation instead of using new technology to measure what's actually happening in the mind."[77]

However, it still remained for Professor Freedman and his co-investigators to (subjectively) interpret the results of the brain scans. "The first interpretation that occurred to me," one of the UCLA neuroscientists said, "is that the Democrats see the 9/11 issue as a good way for Bush to get reelected, and they experience that as a threat." Their enthusiasm overlooks the fact that just because the machines can now locate the source of thought and emotion, they can't tell us anything about why it exists or what it really means.

Stephen Pinker, again: "We are still clueless about how the brain represents the content of our thoughts and feelings. Yes, we may know where jealousy happens—or visual images or spoken words—but 'where' is not the same as 'how.' " *Scientific American* wrote: "Neuroscience . . . has succeeded in unraveling critical chemical and electrical pathways involved in memory, movement and emotion. But reducing the perceptions of a John Coltrane solo or the palette of a Hawaiian sunset to a series of interactions among axons, neurotransmitters, and dendrites still fails to capture what makes an event special. Maybe that's why neuroscience fascinates less than it should."[78] (Axons are the living cables, like wires, that carry electrical impulses to other neurons; dendrites are the treelike spindly branches that grow out of the cell body of the neuron and receive the signals.)

Nevertheless, the smashing victory of biological psychiatry was almost universally endorsed by the end of the 1990s. The following chorus of voices joyously proclaimed its triumph:

> The bases of mental illness are chemical changes in the brain . . . There's no longer any justification for the distinction . . . between mind and body or mental and physical illnesses. Mental illnesses are physical illnesses.
>
> —DAVID SATCHER, U.S. SURGEON GENERAL, 1999 STATEMENT

> All mental processes, even the most complex psychological processes, derive from operations of the brain. The central tenet of this view is that what we commonly call mind is a range of functions carried out by the brain.
>
> —ERIC KANDEL, NOBEL LAUREATE IN PHYSIOLOGY OR MEDICINE, 1998 STATEMENT

> [E]verything in our conscious life, from feeling pains, tickles, and itches to—pick your favorite—feeling the angst of post-industrial man under late capitalism or experiencing the ecstasy of skiing in deep powder—is caused by brain processes.
>
> —JOHN SEARLE, SLUSSER PROFESSOR OF PHILOSOPHY, UNIVERSITY OF CALIFORNIA, BERKELEY, 1995

> "You," your joys and your sorrows, your memories and your ambitions, your sense of personal identity and free will, are in fact no more than the behavior of a vast assembly of nerve cells and their associated molecules. As Lewis Carroll's Alice might have phrased it: "You're nothing but a pack of neurons."
>
> —FRANCIS CRICK, NOBEL LAUREATE IN BIOCHEMISTRY, 1994[79]

The ultimate indicator of our newfound faith in scientific psychiatry may be the mysteriously growing placebo effect. When Columbia

University psychiatrist Timothy Walsh analyzed seventy-five trials of antidepressants conducted between 1981 and 2000, he discovered that the response rate to placebo, which are, of course, nothing more than sugar pills, increased about 7 percent per decade.[80] Simply because people thought they were taking pills, they thought they were going to get better.

I saw the power inherent in biological psychiatry, albeit in an entirely different way. I saw its wonders up close, when it is applied most appropriately to the people who most need its power: people with schizophrenia and bipolar disorder and major depression. A woman named Millie, who looked like a bedraggled Joni Mitchell and who had come to Brooklyn via Dublin in order to claim her throne—in her mind—as a folk rock heroine, was my introduction to the problematic but almost always necessary relationship that people with severe mental illness have with the drugs that simultaneously liberate and imprison them. Through Millie, and eventually hundreds of other patients, I vicariously entered the murky and exotic world of mood stabilizers, SSRIs, benzodiazepines, MAOI inhibitors, and antipsychotics. On a daily basis, I saw the Paxils and Prozacs and Neurontins and Zyprexas and Klonopins and Effexors.

"Do you want to see the device that Scotland Yard inserted into my vagina last night?" Millie asked me in a sort of brogue—her Irishness had washed out somewhat in the decade she'd been in the States—on my first day of work as a case manager at an agency providing housing to people with mental illness. I was in her apartment on a home visit to see how she was doing.

Millie didn't wait for my reply and proceeded to extricate with a shaking hand what looked like a brown twig or a twisted cinnamon stick from a piece of crinkled aluminum foil.

"Here it is! They—Scotland Yard—inserted this into me to track my movements!" she shouted. She cackled, which, bizarrely, set off further chattering and squeaking in the apartment. I looked around and saw the source of the noise—two hamsters in a cage in an utterly deranged-looking sitting room. Everywhere there were cigarette butts and days-old cups of coffee, beat-up guitars, note pages of unintelligible song lyrics, and canvases covered with splatters of yellow, orange, and purple paint. Millie was also painter, and she worked in the Jackson Pollock abstract expressionist tradition, though with even less stability than her mentor.

Millie began charging around the room with the cinnamon stick/brown twig/Scotland Yard device in her hand. On the table next to the hamster cage, there were big bottles of medications with strange names like lithium and Depakote and Prolixin. I checked the dates on the bottles, saw that the bottles were filled with pills, and calculated that she hadn't taken her medications for weeks. Millie, winded now from running laps around the apartment, collapsed into a threadbare armchair, tapestries flung over its back, and smoked a cigarette.

"I tell you one thing: Chrissie Hynde never once had to put up with this shit," she said.

Not knowing how to reply, I asked Millie about the hamsters. All of her responses were nonsensical, the words coming in a huge incomprehensible rush. She appeared to tell me something about having walked the length of Manhattan in her bare feet earlier that day and that she had played basketball with kids in Harlem, which she seemed to believe was a wonderful illustration of racial harmony. (I came to learn that this sort of epic journey was not unusual for her; Millie told me later she had once walked from Scotland to London.) Looking down, I saw that her feet were bleeding. She then stubbed the lit cigarette in her dress. I had seen enough: I told her if she agreed to go to the hospital, I would take care of the hamsters while she was away.

After fifteen minutes of sobs and cries alternating with hysterical laughter and much talk of Scotland Yard and Nazi thought control and John Lennon's murder at the hands of Richard Nixon and vaginal insertion by psychiatrists, Millie said she would go. A few minutes later, we were in a cab headed for Mount Sinai Hospital. "Are you a tuna head or a china bean?" Millie asked the cabdriver. When he didn't reply, she said, "Fuck me! Fuck me! Fuck me, like Tony Blair!" He drove even faster than cabdrivers usually do in Manhattan.

"Do you want to see the device that Hitler inserted into my vagina last night?" Millie asked the psychiatrist in the ER. The doctor, clearly more experienced with mania than I was, emphatically said no. Millie responded by telling the doctor that his breath was bad and that he was a closeted fag. I fully agreed with both of these pronouncements. (This was my first experience with what experienced clinicians call "psychotic insight," the eerie, occasional perspicacity of people completely out of their gourd.)

The next week, when I visited Millie in the hospital, it was immediately apparent she had been put back on her lithium and Depakote and Prolixin. She remembered me vaguely, shyly said hello, and spoke in a gentle and mechanical monotone. She didn't remember anything about her manic episode and being hospitalized and shook her head in quiet embarrassment when I told her, during my weekly visits over the next month, about the scene in her apartment when I first met her. (Eventually, she did remember that I'd asked an awful lot of questions about the hamsters, and she thought that there was something wrong with me.) She was hospitalized for six weeks. Each time I saw her, she was more calm, more shaky, and more flat. She eventually did return to her apartment, to take care of her hamsters and very intermittently and occasionally play guitar and paint like a deranged Jackson Pollock. (I suspected her creative bursts occurred when she stopped taking her meds.) But reliably every year, always in late winter or early spring, there would be an episode, remarkably similar to the one I experienced with her, and then the slow, flat recovery. Ultimately, Millie—not getting the reception she anticipated in New York—took her act back to Ireland, where she is perhaps busking on the streets of Dublin.

You could always tell, though, if Millie was taking her meds. She had a constant tremor in her hand—the lithium tremor, we called it—which I came to see as a symbol of her disabled self: the flat, noncreative, nonvital, deflated Millie, who was nonetheless safe and alive.

I spent the next decade running two housing programs for people with mental illness and then working at two psychiatric shelters for the homeless. Day after day, I saw and handled an endless parade of pills and capsules. They came in all shapes and sizes and colors: big and small and tiny; oblong and circular and square and trapezoidal; mint colored and pale white and faint gray and canary yellow and vibrant purple and lurid pink and soft orange. Depakote smelled nice, like vanilla soda, and Wellbutrin like rotten eggs. Giving out the pills to my clients, I wondered about their origins: who invented them and how, and who named them; where are they manufactured? (As overwhelmingly ingested by Americans as they are, a good portion of drugs are actually manufactured off the U.S. mainland, a fact that Big Pharma keeps quiet. There are now seventy-five plants in India approved to manufacture drugs for the American market, the most of any nation save for the United States itself.[81] Ireland is a key manufacturing site, as is Puerto Rico. Many of Pfizer's major products are made in Puerto Rico. A plant in Barceloneta makes Zoloft and Viagra, and another in Vega Baja makes Lipitor and Neurontin.)[82]

I loved the scientific poetry of some of the names of the drugs, and when I came across a really terrible new name, like a new antipsychotic called Abilify, I resolved that I could do better, and my next career should be as a namer of drugs. Some of the drugs cost $5 for a month's supply, and others $250. Most of my clients were taking three, four, five, six different types of drugs, typically at a cost of $200 to $300 a month.

And my first experience with Millie was in many ways typical. I learned that taking the medications, even for people with terribly disabling illnesses, is to make a Faustian deal. I saw that the drugs sapped people of energy and creativity and had powerful potential side effects (in my experience dizziness, nausea, sweating, massive weight gain, involuntary muscle movements, restlessness, sexual dysfunction, premature onset of diabetes, and in extremely rare cases, death, to name a few). In my experience, for 10 to 20 percent of patients, the medications didn't seem to work at all. Even when they were effective, the pills would sometimes mysteriously stop working for no detectable reason.

I found also that patients' complaints about the side effects of their medications were often overlooked by their doctors and the whole system of care. Psychiatry as a whole has been extraordinarily arrogant and insensitive to what patients have been saying for years: that even when they do their job effectively, the medications have some horrendous side effects.

I recall another very early experience with a patient. Tom and I were walking along a side street on the Lower East Side, on the way to his apartment. Tom had been a promising college student and semiprofessional musician until he developed chronic paranoid schizophrenia. He still played drums a little, and he seemed bored with his psychiatric day program, where he was attending groups such as "Current Events," where the day's headlines were read to patients by earnest social workers.

"Why don't you do some reading of your own?" I suggested.

"Oh, I haven't read anything since I started taking my medications. I have blurred vision a lot and get dizzy when I read," he said.

I shrugged it off at the time. I figured that he had no choice but to take the medications, and if they made his vision blurry, he'd just have to put up with it. These days I am more aware of the full picture—the role of the medications in his overall quality of life. The more I worked with patients, the more I saw both the quantity and misery of the side effects. Among the most common are sweating, extreme sensitivity to heat and sun, sexual uninterest and anorgasmia, dry mouth. Some patients needed their blood drawn regularly to monitor for toxicity (lithium) or low white blood cell counts (Clozaril). A common side effect is called tardive dyskinesia. Tardive dyskinesia is a potentially irreversible condition associated with the first generation of antipsychotics, like Thorazine and Haldol. It comes in the form of involuntary muscle movements, typically facial tics, such as quick spasms of the jaw or tongue, or jerky limb movements, which are sometimes accompanied by grunting or sucking sounds. Not only are these problems uncomfortable and embarrassing, they instantly announce to the rest of the world that the sufferer is a mental patient.

But the worst common side effect, in my observed experience, is akathisia: excessive involuntary movement, or simply put, the inability to sit still. The movements are typically stereotypical motor patterns such as pacing, body rocking, or foot tapping. But the feeling inside the self, as it has been described to me countless times, is the urgent sense of needing to crawl out of one's skin. It is not just bodily movement—it is an internal state, a ceaseless, at times unendurable inner agitation. I have hospitalized people for akathisia. The itchy, crawling restlessness literally drove them crazy.

The worst adverse reaction to antipsychotic drugs is extremely rare but can be lethal. It is called neuroleptic malignant syndrome. I encountered it only once, with another of my clients.

Betty was staring up at me—or so I wanted to believe. The closer I looked I saw that there was nothing registering in her eyes. She was merely looking up, without recognition or comprehension. Her body was covered in sweat, her face pallid, her eyes blank and unmoving. She was hooked up to monitors and what looked to be a million dollars' worth of machines. She had a high fever and couldn't move. Intravenous lines ran into her arms. They treated her initially with cooling blankets, ice packs, cooled fluids, nutrients to replace electrolytes, oxygen and meds to bring down the fever and relax the muscles.

Not knowing what else to do, I held her hand, which by contrast to the rest of her body felt intact and healthy.

In so many ways Betty had been unlucky. She suffered horrendously from the voices that instructed her to kill people. Betty was nothing if not a gentle soul, and killing people was the last thing she wanted to do. The voices in fact made her want to kill herself. The only relief she found was in prayer, and in smoking cigarettes, and in watching her beloved soap operas, and in the Ativan, which relaxed her, and the Haldol, which seemed, at times, to quell the voices; that is, until she almost died while taking Haldol.

Over the weekend, Betty complained of flu symptoms and a high fever to the front desk attendant at the residence. When the fever didn't subside, he called 911 and—without knowing it—saved her life. She was brought to the emergency room, and I saw her the next day, rigged to those machines.

Betty was a victim of neuroleptic malignant syndrome, a rare adverse reaction to antipsychotic drugs. What causes the syndrome isn't clear, but it appears to be related to a blockage of the dopamine receptors in the hypothalamus and spinal cord, among other areas. Symptoms include rigid muscles, extremely high temperatures, sweating, unstable blood pressure, rapid heartbeat, and abnormal increases in the number of white blood cells. While the mortality rate used to be 10 to 30 percent, it is now greatly reduced to perhaps 5 or 10 percent, largely because of better awareness and detection. People with NMS can die of pneuomonia, renal failure, seizures, respiratory failure, and cardiovascular collapse.

Betty didn't die, but she never came all the way back. Although she gradually became conscious, everything wasn't the same as before. She was put on another antipsychotic and closely monitored, but things were never the same. She returned to the residence but it didn't work out. She was slower, dumber, more tentative, and scared. A sort of permanent fuzziness set in, and she couldn't keep the voices at bay. The cigarettes and soap operas didn't matter. She wasn't well. She was moved, as they say, to "a higher level of care," a "more structured" residence, where she could be watched more closely. Even temporarily high body temperatures can lead to brain damage, and the rigidity in the muscles causes them to wear away. Betty was like a boxer after a brutal knockout; she left a part of herself in the ring and in the sweaty sheets of that hospital bed.

Unaware of what happened to people like Millie and Betty, Americans have taken to the drugs en masse. The Prozacs and lithiums and Risperdals and Depakotes and Lexapros and Effexors and Neurontins and Zyprexas now flow into us in copious amounts, an unending cascade of medication swishing and gurgling through our collective bloodstreams.

Nowhere are the stakes higher and consequences more potentially perilous than in the medicating of children. Once considered all but taboo, the provision of psychiatric medications to children and adolescents has become commonplace. While Ritalin (which, incidentally, differs little in its pharmacological profile from cocaine)[83] has been used in moderation for hyperactive children for decades, its use, along with antidepressants and antipsychotics, has gone up exponentially in the last decade.

For so many kids today, the taking of psychiatric drugs is simply part of growing up, no big deal, one of the way stations of youth, just part of the furniture. For good or ill, the stigma has largely been lost. In 2004, a report said that more than a million American kids were taking psychotropic drugs, and 11 million antidepressant prescriptions were written for them.[84] When I asked a troubled teenager, himself taking antidepressants, if he talked about his medication with his peers, many of whom were also taking psychiatric drugs, he said no. "Is that because you're a little embarrassed about it?" I asked. "No, no. It's just not that interesting to anybody . . . Just kind of boring," he said.

The current environment is such that a twenty-one-year-old college student can delineate, with a curious combination of pride, shame, and indifference, the last five years of her life by the drugs she was taking in the pages of *New York* magazine. No longer does one measure out life with coffee spoons, as did T. S. Eliot's Prufrock, but with Adderall and Percocets.

> Winter 2001: Metadate, Dextrostat, Dexedrine Spansules, Adderall XR, Strattera (all attention deficit disorder agents)
>
> Spring 2002–Summer 2003: Adderall XR, Dextrostat, marijuana, Effexor, Zyprexa
>
> Fall 2003: Adderall XR, Dextrostat, Zyprexa, alcohol, marijuana, mushrooms, hash, cocaine
>
> Spring 2004: Adderall XR, Dextrostat, muscle relaxants, Ambien, Abilify

Fall 2004: Adderall XR, Dextrostat, Lexapro

June 2005: Lexapro, lots of Lexapro

August 2005: Lexapro, Lamictal (mood stabilizer), Provigil (attention deficit disorder agent), Wellbutrin, Cymbalta (antidepressant), more Lamictal

January 2007: Lamictal[85]

It turns out that the author had been repeatedly misdiagnosed, as psychotic and ADD and depressed, and floridly overmedicated. Her true diagnosis is bipolar disorder and some personality issues. After all that time being "a teenage drug experiment," as the author called herself, all she needed is what she is getting now—Lamictal, for mood disturbances, and cognitive-behavioral therapy, for her interpersonal problems and her depression.

Nationally, the statistics are simultaneously shocking and, well, numbing. Nearly 1 in 5 psychiatric visits by young people resulted in the prescription of an antipsychotic.[86] Antipsychotic drug use by children and adolescents went up fivefold between 1993 and 2002. Sleeping pill use by youth over age ten increased 85 percent between 2000 and 2004.[87] 25 to 50 percent of kids at a typical summer camp take daily prescription medications. Allergy and asthma drugs are the most common, but psychiatric agents are so prevalent that "nurses who dispense them no longer try to avoid stigma by pretending they are vitamins." There's even a company, CampMeds, which prepackages an entire summer's worth of medications for campers in shrink-wrapped packets.[88]

So common are the drugs for children and adults that in 2003 an article appeared in *Time* about a nationwide survey showing that "U.S. rivers and streams are tainted with, among other things, pesticides, antibiotics and even common drugs such as aspirin and Prozac, flushed down drains and out into the water supply."[89]

Although the concentrations are very low, scientists don't yet know if even very low levels are safe. Indeed, the discovery of Prozac in the water is a common enough finding. You could even say we're swimming in Prozac, or at least the fish are. Bryan Brooks, a Baylor University toxicologist, tested three species of fish—bluegill, black crappie, and channel catfish—downstream from a water-treatment plant in northern Texas, and found the active ingredients of Prozac and Zoloft in their brains and livers. "We detected all of the compounds in every tissue of the fish we tested," Brooks told the annual meeting of the Geological Society of America.[90] Another toxicologist subsequently discovered that low levels of Prozac, Paxil, Zoloft, and Celexa cause developmental lags in fish and in frogs.[91] Traces of Prozac and Valium were also reported to have been found in Lake Mead, the Nevada reservoir that supplies drinking water to Los Angeles and Phoenix.[92] (One wonders if this extra supply of antidepressants explains why the citizens of those cities have a reputation for being particularly laid-back and mellow.)

It's a situation that would have made the late physician-novelist Walker Percy very unhappy. Well, actually, proud and unhappy. Proud because he predicted the omnipresence of psychiatric drugs in his last novel, *The Thanatos Syndrome*, published in 1987, the year before Prozac appeared on the market. And unhappy because it was a situation that he would have despaired over. Hence the title, from Freud: Thanatos, signifying aggression, evil, the death instinct, is the opposite of Eros, which refers to libidinal energy, or the "life force."

In the novel's opening pages, Dr. Thomas More, a psychiatrist who used to be a visionary scientist but now considers himself just an old-fashioned "psyche-iatrist"—a "physician of the soul, one of the last survivors in a horde of Texas brain mechanics, MIT neurone [*sic*] circuitrists"—is released from federal prison after two years of incarceration for selling prescription amphetamines at a truck stop. He returns to his practice (where he is both a patient and a doctor) in his hometown of Feliciana, Louisiana, and notices that something has changed in his patients: "In each, there has occurred a sloughing away of the old terrors, worries, rage, a shedding of guilt like last year's snakeskin."[93] But while their troubles are now obscured and under control, they have been replaced by a dull, feckless, and vast empty-headedness. All of his patients' foibles and idiosyncrasies—all that made them interesting and human and alive—have been removed. Dr. More investigates old enemies, the "Director of the Quality-of-Life Division of the Federal Euthanasia Program" and the head of the computer division of the nuclear plant (both of whom were involved in sending him to prison), and discovers they have enacted a brilliant bit of social engineering for the betterment of the populace. They have been putting "Heavy Sodium" in the drinking water to numb out the population and make it, supposedly, happy and content. Dr. More uncovers the conspiracy, stops the placement of Heavy Sodium in the water supply, and thereby returns his patients to normal—their vitality, as well as their troubles, restored. In the place of Heavy Sodium, Dr. More calls for an authentic *unmedicated* human experience, however painful it may at times be.

While the residents of Feliciana, victims of a conspiracy, had no choice in being medicated (though I think Percy would argue that most Americans, bombarded as they have been by Zoloft ads in the last decade, have had little choice themselves), Percy presciently identified the first of the dual tragedies of biological psychiatry: its indiscriminate use by anyone who even thinks they have a problem. And although Percy predicted the problems with the overuse of antidepressants, it has played out, over the last fifteen years, in an even darker way than he described.

The problem with our full-on embrace of biological psychiatry is that it is terribly premature. The truth is that we are only in the very early and primitive stages of understanding how the brain works and what alters its functioning. Somewhere along the way we seemed to have misplaced the notion that, at this stage of our scientific evolution at least, the brain's capacity to understand itself is minimal. The task is daunting. For the record, there are more than 100 billion neurons in the human brain. Each neuron is connected to hundreds and thousands of other neurons, and each neuron can fire hundreds of times a second to other neurons across synapses. Altogether there are 100 trillion synapses through which the electrical and neurochemical messages flow. The connections are just about infinite. All of this activity happens within the confines of a three- to four-pound object. And the brain isn't even mainly composed of neurons. Ninety percent of the cells in the brain are actually *not* neurons. They are glial cells, which provide nutrition and protection to the neurons. Glial cells have historically been overlooked in brain research, but there is mounting evidence and a growing awareness that the glia have critical and active roles in many brain functions, and dysfunctions.[94]

The brain is the most complicated object in the universe. Nobel Prize–winning psychiatrist Eric Kandel has written, "In fact, we are only beginning to understand the simplest mental functions in biological terms; we are far from having a realist neurobiology of clinical syndromes."[95] Neuroscientist Torsten Wiesel, another Nobelist, scoffed at the hubris involved in naming the 1990s "The Decade of the Brain," by presidential proclamation. "Foolish," he called it. "We need at least a century, maybe even a millennium" to comprehend the brain. "We still don't know how *C. elegans* works," he said, referring to a small worm that is often used by scientists to study molecular and cell biology.[96] In my travels in the neuro world, I have consistently found that the elite scientists are surprisingly modest about how little we know about the brain, despite spectacular progress in recent decades. It is the midlevel scientists who are prone to making exalted claims about the certainty and sophistication of our present knowledge.

To this day, no one knows exactly how the drugs work. The etiology of depression remains an enduring scientific mystery, with entirely new ways of understanding the disease—or *diseases*, as what we think of as "depression" now is probably dozens of discrete disease entities—emerging constantly. While serotonin has *something* to do with depression, the relationship is not a simple nor a well-understood one. No deficiencies in the serotonin system have consistently been reported among depressed people; in fact, no simple one-to-one relationship between any psychiatric disorder and a single neurotransmitter has ever been proven.[97] While the SSRIs do indeed act on serotonin regulation in the brain, allowing the neurotransmitter to linger a little longer in the synapses, the changes that the drug ultimately exerts on the brain are entirely unclear. As an indicator of how little we know, it is striking that one of the more popular antidepressants in Europe, tianeptine, is a serotonin reuptake *enhancer*—it has the opposite effect of the SSRIs, allowing less serotonin to flow between the synapses. And yet it, too, can be an effective antidepressant!

The flimsiness of the entire enterprise was brought home to me in devastating fashion in a conversation with Elliot Valenstein, a leading neuroscientist at the University of Michigan and author of three highly regarded and influential books on psychopharmacology and the history of psychiatry. I was talking to Dr. Valenstein about why all psychiatric drugs address only a very small proportion of the neurotransmitters that are thought to exist. Virtually all psychiatric drugs deal with only 4 neurotransmitters: dopamine and serotonin, most commonly, and also norepinephrine, and GABA (gamma-aminobutyric acid). While no one knows exactly how many neurotransmitters there are in the human brain—indeed, even how a neurotransmitter is defined exactly can be a matter of debate—there are at least 100, perhaps 125.

So I asked Dr. Valenstein, "Why do all the drugs all deal with the same brain chemicals? Is it because those four neurotransmitters are the ones understood to be most implicated with mood and thought regulation—i.e., the stuff of psychiatric disorders?"

"It's entirely a historical accident," he said. "The first psychiatric drugs were stumbled upon in the dark, completely serendipitously. No one, least of all the people who discovered them, had any idea how they worked. It was only later that the science caught up and provided evidence that those drugs influence those particular neurotransmitters. After that, all subsequent drugs were 'copycats' of the originals—and all of them regulating only those same four neurotransmitters. There have not been any new radically different paradigms of drug action that have been developed." Indeed, while by 1997 one hundred drugs had been designed to treat schizophrenia, all of them resembled the original, Thorazine, in their mechanism of action.[98]

"So," I asked Dr. Valenstein, "if the first drugs that were discovered dealt with a different group of neurotransmitters, then all the drugs in use today would involve an entirely different set of neurotransmitters?"

"Yes," he said.

"In other words, there are more than a hundred neurotransmitters, some of which could have vital impact on psychiatric syndromes, yet to be explored?" I asked.

"Absolutely," Dr. Valenstein said. "It's all completely arbitrary."

Indeed one of the basic tenets of biological psychiatry, that depression is a result of a deficit in serotonin (or the "monoamine theory of depression," as it is known in the scientific literature), has proven prematurely seductive to psychiatric practitioners and patients alike. When the monoamine theory emerged in the 1960s, it gave the biologically minded practitioners of psychiatry what they had long been craving—a clean, decisive, scientific theory to help bring the field in line with the rest of medicine. For patients, too, the serotonin hypothesis was enormously appealing. It not only provided the soothing clarity of a physical explanation of their maladies, it absolved them of responsibility for their illness, and to some degree, their behavior. Because, after all, who's responsible for a chemical imbalance?

Unfortunately, from the very start, there was a massive contradiction at the heart of the monoamine theory. Whatever it is that SSRIs do to change brain chemistry, it happens almost immediately after they are ingested. The neurochemical changes are quick. However, SSRIs typically take weeks, even months, to have any therapeutic influence. Why the delay? No one had any explanation, until the late 1990s, when Ronald Duman, a researcher at Yale, showed that antidepressants *actually grow brain cells* in the hippocampus, a part of the brain associated with memory and mood regulation.[99] Such a development would have been viewed as preposterous even a decade earlier; one of the central dogmas of brain science for more than a century has been that the adult brain is incapable of producing new neurons, a belief that has been disproved by Duman and a host of other well-regarded scientists. Duman believes that it takes weeks or months to build up a critical mass of the new brain cells in order to exert a healing process in the brain.

While Duman's explanation for the mechanism of action of the SSRIs remains controversial, a consensus is building that most likely

SSRIs initiate a series of complex changes, involving many neurotransmitters, that alter the functioning of the brain at the cellular and molecular levels. The emerging truth appears to be that the SSRIs may be only the necessary first step of a "cascade" of brain changes that occur long after, and well "downstream," of serotonin alterations. The frustrating truth is that depression, and all mental illnesses, are incredibly complicated and poorly understood diseases, involving many neurotransmitters, many genes, and an intricate, infinite, dialectical dance between experience and biology. One of the leading serotonin researchers, Jeffrey Meyer, of the University of Toronto, summed up the misplaced logic of the monoamine hypothesis: "There is a common misunderstanding that serotonin is low during clinical depression. It mostly comes from the fact that many antidepressants raise serotonin. This is a bit like saying pneumonia is an illness of low antibiotics because we treat pneumonia with antibiotics."[100] Correlation with serotonin is not necessarily causation by serotonin.[101]

Furthermore, the monoamine system comprises only a small percent of the neurons in the brain. The largest regulatory systems in the brain are the glutamate and GABA (gamma-aminobutyric acid) systems. Glutamate excites neurons and induces activity, whereas GABA inhibits neurons.[102] Gerard Sanacora at Yale is pursuing research into these neurotransmitter systems. What he finds there could produce a far more holistic and comprehensive understanding of and treatment for depression.

For the exaggerations and aggressive marketing on the part of the drug companies, and for all the hasty embrace of biological psychiatry, it is nonetheless true that millions of people are taking antidepressants and psychiatric drugs every night, of their own accord. No one is directly forcing them to do so. For years now, tens of millions of Americans have willingly taken the pills, put them in their mouths, and swallowed. Those one in six residents of Winterset, while manipulated, are perfectly happy going to the Montross Pharmacy to get their monthly supply of Lexapro.

What does this say about us? What does it say about how we, as a culture, live now and how we choose to solve problems? What does it say about how we view our emotions? What does it say about our psyches, and our souls? In other words, *why* did it happen?

I suspect that the answer has something to do with misery.

CHAPTER FOUR

American Misery

I am thinking of those millions and millions of Medicated Americans—that vast discontented army, those 11 percent of American women and 5 percent of American men who are taking antidepressants.

These Medicated Americans are looking at themselves in the mirror. I can see these Medicated Americans, these millions and millions of putatively psychiatrically distressed people standing alone in their bathrooms late at night, looking at their faces in the bathroom mirror. It is Sunday night. The Medicated American is getting ready for bed. Monday morning and its attendant pressures—the rush to get out of the house, the long commute, the bustle of the office—loom. The Medicated American stands alone, in the middle of the suddenly quiet night, contemplating this.

The Medicated American—let us call her Julie, and let us place her in Winterset, Iowa—opens the cabinet of the bathroom vanity, removes a medicine bottle, and taps one, two, three pills into her palm. She fills a glass of water, places the colorful pills in her mouth, and swallows. The little pills, which could be any one of thirty available drugs used as antidepressants—Prozac or Zoloft or Paxil or Celexa or Lexapro or Luvox or BuSpar or Nardil or Elavil or Sinequan or Pamelor or Serzone or Desyrel or Norpramin or Tofranil or Adapin or Vivactil or Ludiomil or Endep or Parnate or Remeron—make a slight, not unpleasant flutter as they pass down her throat. Julie examines her face in the mirror and sighs. She tightens the cap, places the bottle back in the cabinet, puts the glass by the sink, and thinks abstractly of the pills settling in her stomach. Already they are probably starting to dissolve and break up. What happens after that, she doesn't really know.

Staring at her face, Julie hopes that by some Monday morning in the future—if not tomorrow morning, then some mythical and brilliant and shimmering Monday morning a month from now, or two months from now, or three—the pills will have worked some kind of inexorable magic. Corrected a chemical imbalance, or something, as the Zoloft commercial had said. "Zoloft, a prescription medicine, can help. It works to correct chemical imbalances in the brain," the voiceover on the ad had intoned. Julie didn't know she had a chemical imbalance and doesn't actually know what one is, and it had never really occurred to her that she could have a mental illness (could she?), but she does hope, fervently, that her life will become a little easier, a little less stressed, and more smoothed out—soon. She hopes, desperately, that the pills will make her feel better—that the little white powder hidden in the green capsule will dissolve in her stomach, enter her bloodstream, travel to her brain, and do something—do something to her serotonin, she thinks. Brushing her teeth, she hopes that one day she will simply feel better.

If statistics serve, we know a number of things about the Medicated American. We know that there's a very good chance she does not even have a psychiatric diagnosis. A study of antidepressant use in private health insurance plans found that a majority of those prescribed antidepressants received no psychiatric diagnosis or any mental health care beyond the prescription of the drug.[1] We know, first of all, that she is female: twice as many psychiatric drugs are prescribed for women as men.[2] Remarkably, in 2002, more than one in three doctor's office visits by women involved the prescription of an antidepressant, either for a new prescription or the maintenance of an existing one.[3]

We know that her antidepressants were likely not prescribed by a psychiatrist: most antidepressants are now prescribed by family doctors.[4] We know that Julie in Iowa was far more likely to ask her doctor for an antidepressant after having seen it advertised on TV or in print, and when Julie asked for her antidepressant, her doctor was likely to comply with the request, even if he or she felt ambivalent about the choice of drug or diagnosis.[5] And the requests themselves are very common; one in five Americans have asked their doctor for a drug after they've seen it advertised.[6]

It's extremely unlikely that the doctor spent a whole lot of time talking to Julie about the nature of the drugs, the common side effect profiles, and the remote but potentially dangerous side effects. Research has confirmed what we have all experienced—doctors don't do all that much talking when they prescribe a drug. Based on taped sessions, a study showed that when prescribing a new medicine, two-thirds of doctors said nothing to the patient about how long to take the medication, and almost half did not indicate the dosage amount and frequency. Only about a third of the time did doctors talk about adverse side effects.[7] This is no doubt a function of the pressure to process patients, but it's also a function of old-school medical arrogance and aloofness from patient concerns. The doctor is in charge and the patient complies without creating too much of a fuss. In the case of antidepressants, failure to review possible side effects and to monitor the patient's progress in the weeks and months after starting the drugs is deeply irresponsible. *The Journal of the American Medical Association* states, "The risk of suicidal behavior is increased in the first month after starting antidepressants, especially during the first one to nine days."[8]

There's no longer any need to deal with an actual physician: all these drugs are readily available, with a few clicks and a ready credit card, at Web sites like www.anxietydisorders.biz and www.drugsupplier.biz. Anyone who gets e-mail receives these sort of solicitations weekly, if not daily:

SPAM best price$ for top qulity [*sic*] meds:

Visit our new online pharmacy store and save up too [*sic*] 85%

Todays [*sic*] special offers: VIAGRA FOR AS LOW AS $1.62 PER DOSE

—All popular drugs are available—Free shipping worlwide [*sic*]

—No Doctor Visits

—No Prescriptions

—100% Customer Satisfaction

Click here to visit our new pharmacy store.

Have a nice day.

We further know that Julie's managed-care insurance company was more than happy to cover the prescription, especially if it meant that they didn't have to pay for therapy, which Julie was less and less likely, and less and less able, to pursue. As noted, the vast majority of antidepressant prescriptions are written by family doctors—an unsurprising fact given that there are only about forty-five thousand psychiatrists in the country. As a result, after starting antidepressants and taking them for three months, three-quarters of adults and over half of children do not see a doctor or therapist specifically for mental heath care.[9] Another report found that only 20 percent of people who take antidepressants have any kind of follow-up appointment to monitor the medication.[10]

Between 1987 and 1997, while the rate of pharmacological treatment for depression doubled, the number of psychotherapy visits for depression decreased.[11] These days, only about 3 percent of the population receives therapy from a psychiatrist, psychologist, or social worker.[12] What has happened is that in the last twenty years, as insurers have paid for psychotropic medications, they have compensated for the extra costs by "carving out" the rest of mental health care—inpatient stays, intensive outpatient, residential services, and psychotherapy—from their general benefits package. Those "specialty services" are managed by subcontractors, "managed behavioral health care" groups, which in my experience have a reputation for watching expenses and denying services with even more vigilance and ruthlessness than general managed care.[13] Talk to almost any social worker or psychologist, and they will tell you, probably for longer than you want to hear, how brutal managed care has been to their practice. Reimbursement rates have systematically been cut or have not kept up with inflation, causing a number of psychotherapists to leave the field. *The New York Times* ran a story about a social worker who took on work as a seamstress on the side in order to get by.[14] Denying claims for arbitrary reasons, cutting back on the number of authorized sessions, paying late: these are all standard fare. More than these actual hassles, what is so unsettling to many mental health professionals is the general message of managed care: that the work they are doing is not consequential or clinically robust. The era of managed care has amounted to an ongoing assault on the practice of psychotherapy. (The first psychiatric benefit in a health insurance plan, incidentally, was implemented on September 1, 1951, by Kaiser Permanente in Oakland, California. Services were provided at a small inpatient hospital and outpatient clinic in San Francisco. One of the chief architects of the plan happened to be the psychologist Timothy Leary, of—much later—LSD and "Turn On, Tune In, and Drop Out" fame.)[15]

"Managed-care plans along with employers have been reluctant to pay the cost of ongoing psychotherapy," said physician-author Timothy B. McCall in his commentary on National Public Radio's *Marketplace*. "Even patients with serious disorders that stem from such things as childhood sexual abuse are being limited to just a few visits. That's if they are being seen by a therapist at all . . . The only area of mental health coverage that employers and HMOs seem interested in funding is drug therapy. They'd rather just throw Prozac, or better yet, some generic substitute costing pennies a pill, at mental health problems."[16] The strong likelihood is that the nightly fluttering of the two or three pills down her throat will be the extent of Julie's "mental health treatment."

Most significantly, we can be assured that the odds are strong that Julie does not have a severe and persistent mental illness, such as schizophrenia, bipolar disorder, severe forms of depression, or obsessive-compulsive disorder. According to the U.S. Surgeon General's *Report on Mental Health*, only 2.6 percent of American adults have such entrenched conditions, which are treated—for those who receive treatment—by antidepressants, antipsychotics, mood stabilizers, and antianxiety agents. Meanwhile, more than 10 percent of American women are taking antidepressants alone. Most likely, Julie's complaints fall into "that considerable gray area between feelings and behaviors that constitute a disorder and those of a similar nature that are not severe or specific enough to merit a diagnosis," as *Psychiatric News*, a journal of the American Psychiatric Association, put it. "A few examples: shyness vs. social phobic disorder, a gloomy disposition vs. dysthymic disorder, dissatisfaction with one's appearance or sexual performance vs. body dysmorphic or hypoactive sexual desire disorder, getting upset when things go wrong vs. adjustment disorder."[17] And that's if the prescribing doctor even gives a diagnosis. An analysis of data on patients insured by private health insurance companies found that 42 percent of users were not given any clearly identified mental-health or even off-label indication when they were prescribed antidepressants. In other words, the doctor gave no psychiatric reason for writing the prescription.[18]

While SSRIs were first approved as treatment for clinical depression, other uses were steadily added during the course of the 1990s: indications came, one after the other, for obsessive-compulsive disorder, eating disorders, anxiety, and premenstrual dysphoric disorder (a severe form of premenstrual syndrome). The drugs were also used for paraphilias, sexual compulsions, and body dysmorphic disorder. With each new utilization, the market got bigger, lines between distress and disease got blurrier, and the drugs began to be prescribed for problems beyond those indicated by the FDA. As a result, a good portion of Americans are now taking SSRIs for non-FDA-approved uses, termed "off-label" prescriptions. A University of Georgia study found that three-quarters of people prescribed antidepressant drugs receive the medications for a reason not approved by the Food and Drug Administration.[19] This practice is legal and intended to give physicians the flexibility to prescribe the drugs that are best suited to their patients' needs. The problem is that "most off-label drug mentions have little or no scientific support," said study co-author Jack Fincham, of the University of Georgia College of Pharmacy. "And when I say most, it's like 70 to 75 percent. Many patients have no idea that this goes on and just assume that the physician is writing a prescription for their indication."[20] Off-label prescribing for drugs in general has soared, nearly doubling in the period between 1997 and 2003.[21] One of the taglines used in the ads for Zoloft tacitly acknowledges the never-ending applicability of its formulary—"Zoloft—#1 for Millions of Reasons."

So, if not for a serious mental illness, what exactly is Julie taking the antidepressants for? There are a couple of alternatives. First, there is the catchall term *depression.* Depression, once considered a rare disease associated usually with elderly women, is overwhelmingly the mental health diagnosis of choice of our time. About 40 percent of mental health visits are for depression, according to the Centers for Disease Control.[22] As perhaps America's most influential academic psychologist, Martin Seligman, has stated: "If you're born around World War I, in your lifetime the prevalence of depression is about 1 percent. If you're born around World War II the lifetime prevalence of depressions seemed to be about 5 percent. If you were born starting in the 1960s, the lifetime prevalence seemed to be between 10 percent and 15 percent, and this is with lives incomplete." That's at least a tenfold increase in the amount of depression in two generations. Furthermore, the age of onset of the first depressive episode has moved up dramatically. A generation or two ago, the onset of depression occurred on average at age thirty-four or thirty-five; in recent studies, the mean age for the first bout of depression was fourteen years old.[23]

It's as if from the early 1990s on (nicely coinciding with the mass penetration of Prozac), we have been living in the Age of Depression—just as Valium arrived in, or helped create, the Age of Anxiety. As always, the diagnoses follow the pills available to treat them. But in contemporary America, it has been broadly accepted for some time that everybody, at some level, is depressed at least some of the time. We all relate to some aspect of depression in its broad iteration, particularly when it's a dull late afternoon in March, the snow is falling again, and a headache is coming on. Many aspects of life are undeniably tedious, annoying, vaguely painful—traffic jams, news headlines, bank errors. As Americans have become more aware of their feelings in the last three therapy-oriented decades, it has become acceptable and eminently appropriate to say, when someone asks how you are feeling (particularly if it's late March), "a little depressed." Or to respond to the query, "How was the movie the other day?": "A little depressing." Or to say, in response to "How did you feel about last year's minuscule raise?": "Depressed." The author (and depression sufferer) William Styron wrote that the word "has slithered innocuously through the language like a slug, leaving little trace of its intrinsic malevolence and preventing, by its very insipidity, a general awareness of the horrible intensity of the disease when out of control."[24]

But to anyone reasonably experienced in the mental health field, there is depression, and then there is Depression. The first type of depression is a terribly broad and bland term, indicating "the blues," "feeling down," "bummed out," "in the dumps," "low," "a little tired," "not quite myself," each a standard part of the daily human predicament. That "blacker form" of depression, major depressive disorder, is what Styron is referring to when he uses terms like *malevolent*, *horrible*, and *out of control.* Major depression is a harrowing and indisputably profound and serious medical condition. To confuse the two—depression with Depression—is to compare a gentle spring rain to an unrelenting and vengeful typhoon. A true diagnosis of major depression involves some combination of most of the following: inability to feel pleasure of any kind whatsoever, loss of interest in everything, extreme self-hatred or guilt, inability to concentrate or to do the simplest things, sleeping all the time or not being able to sleep at all, dramatic weight gain or loss, and wanting to kill yourself or actually trying to kill yourself. Truly depressed people do not smile or laugh; they may not talk; they are not fun to be with; they do not wish to be visited; they may not eat and have to be fed with feeding tubes so as not to die; and they exude a palpable and monstrous sense of pain. It is a thing unto itself, an undeniably physical and medical affliction, and *not,* as the psychiatrist Paul McHugh writes, "just the dark side of human emotion."[25]

One feels their anguish at a primal, physiological level. "Very often, patients with major depression will say the emotional pain they feel is worse than the pain of any physical illness," says Dr. John J. Mann, chief of neuroscience at Columbia University.[26] There is absolutely nothing good, or worthwhile, about the suffering. It is literally unbearable, insufferable, insupportable. Many depressed people really, really want to die, and thinking about dying, or planning their death, takes up a great deal of their time. So horrific is the incapacitation that the highest risk of suicide actually comes when people are feeling slightly better. In the throes of an episode, depressed patients are too dissipated to even muster the energy to kill themselves. Even highly articulate chroniclers of depression are stumped when attempting to describe the depths of pain: a writer as prodigiously elegant as Styron is reduced to using the word *indescribable.* As for the notion that major depression is associated with increased creativity: if one is truly depressed, one doesn't pick up a pen, a brush, a camera, or conduct a scientific experiment. One lies in bed, too ill to even moan. The only thing one might pick up is a razor blade after feeling slightly better. I do, however, believe that some small minority of people, assuming they survive a significant depression with their faculties intact, are bothered enough by things as they are that they are then motivated to create something new. As H. L. Mencken wrote about artists in general, they feel an itch that other people don't feel. The notion of suggesting that sufferers "snap out of it," "pull themselves up by their bootstraps," "face the day," all perfectly appropriate ministrations for the other type of depression, is ludicrous and even cruel. It is the equivalent of imploring "Can't you do better?" to terminal cancer patients or advising a person right after a heart attack to "get back on your feet."

I thought I knew the difference between the blues and major depression until I saw the disease in its full and malicious force. Any number of times I have witnessed heretofore vibrant, functioning people transformed into sobbing, quivering wrecks. Truly depressed people shake physically, are unable to get out of bed, and exude a profound heaviness or lifelessness, exhibiting a sort of death in life. For all of its efficacy, at this point psychotherapy and other psychosocial approaches won't make much of a difference. There is simply not that much to say. The only treatments are hospitalization, supervision, rest, quiet, sedatives, sleep medications, an appropriate level of antidepressants, and electroconvulsive therapy. Despite its side effects (such as short-term memory loss), electroconvulsive therapy remains the single most effective treatment for major depression.

The best descriptions of the torments of depression I have encountered happen to be centuries old, well predating our more sophisticated clinical terminology, our symptom lists, and our billing codes. In an 1806 diary, a Nova Scotia evangelist vividly described his personal psychic torments. The writer, Henry Alline, would not have viewed his anguishes as an episode of depression at all—perhaps a spiritual crisis or a bout of religious melancholia. Nonetheless, it is major depression that he describes:

> Everything I saw seemed to be a burden to me; the earth seemed accursed for my sake: all trees, plants, rocks, hills, and vales seemed to be dressed in mourning and groaning, under the weight of the curse, and everything around me seemed to be conspiring my ruin . . . I had now so great a sense of the vanity and emptiness of all things here below, that I knew the whole world could not possibly make me happy . . . When I waked in the morning, the first thought would be, Oh, my wretched soul, what shall I do, where shall I go? . . . when I have seen birds flying over my head, [I] have often thought within myself, Oh, that I could fly away from my danger and distress! Oh, how happy should I be, if I were in their place![27]

And then there is Emily Dickinson, the poet laureate of melancholy, writing in the mid-1800s:

I felt a Funeral, in my Brain,
And Mourners to and fro
Kept treading—treading—till it seemed
That Sense was breaking through—

And when they all were seated,
A Service, like a Drum—
Kept beating—beating—till I thought
My Mind was going numb—

And then I heard them lift a Box
And creak across my Soul
With those same Boots of Lead, again,
Then Space—began to toll,

As all the Heavens were a Bell,
And Being, but an Ear,
And I, and Silence, some strange Race
Wrecked, solitary, here

To anyone who has truly suffered from mental illness, there is no better seven-word description of the chill and fear and suffering than "I felt a funeral in my brain."

But until such time as there are some kinds of biomarkers in psychiatry—physiological tests (such as genetic testing, brain scans, potentially relevant data from blood and hormone tests, et cetera) upon which to rationally base a diagnosis—there is no truly objective, rigorous, "scientific" way to differentiate Depression from depression, as well as other severe mental illnesses, from their related but hugely less debilitating cousins. Work toward the establishment of biomarkers is currently being undertaken. While the use of such biomarkers is probably decades away, and many of the tests will be subtle and highly subject to interpretation, the advent of these technologies could greatly enhance the validity of psychiatric diagnosis and treatment. Their use in everyday clinical practice to guide treatment and drug choices will remove us from the diagnostic gray areas that the drug companies have so successfully exploited. For now, however, the difference between Depression and depression is a matter of completing symptom checklists and clinical judgment.

But I can say that a highly experienced and expert clinician can instantly identify major depression when they see it. It is immediately detectable to people who know what they are doing. It is an advanced physiological state of despair that one can see in the patient's eyes, in their slow movements, in the sense that they are in physical pain, in the fact that they often have not slept or eaten for days, in their lack of humor, in the proximity of death and dying in their conversation (that is, if the patient is talking) and surrounding their very presence, in the obvious fact that they do not presently want to be awake, or alive. There is no covering up; they exude naked and pure pain, like a wounded animal. There is absolutely no pretending that everything is okay. All pretense of normalcy goes out the window. As a particularly insightful social worker once said to me, after we had been struggling for six months to manage a facility for people suffering from schizophrenia: "You know, the difference between people with severe mental illness and the rest of us is that they simply cannot put their problems in a box. All of us have problems, but most of us are able to compartmentalize those problems and get on with our lives. People with severe mental illness can't do that." As unscientific as that sounds, it's about the best way of broadly defining and distinguishing severe mental illness from its benign and watered-down versions that I've yet encountered.

In other words, if Julie were actually suffering from major depression, she probably wouldn't be watching the Super Bowl, wouldn't be having friends around for a party, and wouldn't be going to work anytime soon. She probably wouldn't be getting out of bed.

But that doesn't stop the universal usage of the diagnosis, such that, according to the Centers for Disease Control, doctors reported 21 million ambulatory office visits to physicians for "depression" in 2003.[28] Proper screening for major depression requires a detailed interview and familiarity with the ten major symptoms of the disease. The vast majority of primary care doctors have neither the time nor the expertise (nor the interest, perhaps) to do this screening. Studies have shown that primary care doctors make the correct diagnosis only about two-thirds of the time.[29] And even among trained interviewers administering the SCID, or Structured Clinical Interview for the DSM series, the self-proclaimed "gold standard" of psychiatric diagnosis, the chances of two independent evaluators both arriving at a diagnosis of major depression for the same patient has been reported at only about 80 percent.[30] All of this is to say that, while Julie may have received a diagnosis of major depression in order to receive her Prozac or Paxil (and for her doctor to be reimbursed for the visit), it is unlikely that she *has* major depression.

What modern psychiatry has done, I am convinced, is to conflate and confuse the two, Depression and depression. David Healy calls it a "wholesale creation of depression on so extraordinary and unwarranted a scale" so as "to raise grave questions about whether the pharmaceutical and other health care companies are more wedded to making profits from health than contributing to it."[31] To treat the moderately ill before the severely ill sets a terrible precedent. It seems to go against the basic medical ethic: triage. You treat the worst affected people first.

The second likely mechanism by which Julie got her Prozac was by receiving a clinical diagnosis for what is in fact a troublesome life situation, such as divorce, the pressures of the workplace, or adjusting to change. In other words, psychological distress, but not mental illness. A 2007 study showed that about one in four people who appear to be depressed are in fact dealing with the aftermath of a recent emotional blow, like the end of a marriage, the loss of a job, or the collapse of a business.[32] "Serious Psychological Distress" is a measure used by the federal Substance Abuse and Mental Health Services Administration. They find it highly prevalent: an average of 9 percent of Americans report having experienced psychological distress in a given year. Interestingly, psychological distress is far more common in the western and southern states (the red states, mainly) than in the Northeast and Midwest. States with particularly high rates are Arkansas, Kansas, Kentucky, Missouri, Oklahoma, South Carolina, Utah, West Virginia, Wyoming, and the one exception to the geographical rule, Rhode Island. The least stressed-out state, predictably, is Hawaii.[33]

Each successive edition of the DSM (the *Diagnostic and Statistical Manual of Mental Disorders*) has proclaimed an ever-increasing number of diagnoses that cover an ever-widening terrain of normal, if painful, human behavior. DSM-I, which was published in 1952 and heavily influenced by William Menninger's taxonomy of disorders produced during World War II, covered sixty-two diagnoses. DSM-IV, which came out in 1994, had over three hundred. (On the shelf, DSM-I is a little pamphlet, while DSM-IV is a thick reference volume weighing in at about three pounds.) The next version, DSM-V, due in 2012, will likely introduce even more. (The first attempt to record and classify psychiatric data in the United States was during the 1840 census, in which the frequency of "idiocy/insanity" was recorded. By the 1880 census, seven types of insanity had been codified: mania, melancholia, monomania [obsession or paranoia], paresis [general or partial paralysis], dementia, dipsomania [alcoholism], and epilepsy.)[34]

It is only fairly recently that such problems of living were considered to be in the purview of psychiatry at all. With some exceptions (upper-class neurotics on Freud's couch), the original charge of psychiatry was to treat the severely mentally ill. (And even then, Freud concentrated on cases with a high degree of pathology.) Psychiatry's original efforts, however primitive and misguided, were focused on creating asylums for people unable to live without constant supervision and support. In what I think is a tragic misstep, psychiatry has chosen to take on all the problems of the world. It has chosen to take on alienation, which is a terribly murky area in which to do business. As Karl Menninger, William's brother and also one of psychiatry's most influential figures, wrote in the boundless glow of the 1960s: "Nothing of human concern is really outside psychiatry. So in one sense I have no hobbies. They are all part of my work."[35] One would think that attempting to alleviate the suffering of severe mental illnesses such as bipolar disorder, major depression, and schizophrenia would be a challenging enough task. But, in a clear case of a business expanding its market base, much of psychiatry has abandoned its initial mission to serve the severely mentally ill and gravitated toward the more lucrative "psychoneuroses," as the historian of psychiatry Edward Shorter has put it. Shorter contends that this shift is entirely defensive and self-serving, a response to increasing competition from nonmedical mental health professionals like social workers and psychologists, who began treating the "worried well," "garden-variety" neurotics in the 1970s.

As the SSRI revolution has worn on, it has become increasingly clear that *the wrong people are taking the medications.* This is a scenario that is now manifestly true of most of the people taking these drugs, who may be unhappy, even mildly depressed, but whose conditions are not disabling enough to add up to an illness. Carl Elliott has written that, not long after their introduction, "clinicians soon started to use SSRIs to treat social phobia, obsessive-compulsive disorder, premenstrual dysphoric disorder, eating disorders, paraphilias, sexual compulsions, body dysmorphic disorder, and generalized anxiety disorder. With each new disorder came a new market of potential antidepressant users: uptight Americans, melancholy Americans, weight-obsessed Americans, shy and lonely Americans sitting at home on the couch, watching cable TV . . . As long as the SSRIs were being prescribed for serious depression, their benefits clearly outweighed the risks. But nobody seriously believes that SSRIs are prescribed only or even largely for serious depression anymore."[36] As Edward Shorter has argued, the threshold of what constitutes a psychiatric illness has been dramatically lowered. What was once viewed as angst or distress has been reframed in psychological, psychiatric, and medicalized terms. In shifting to the more common and "more lucrative" psychoneuroses, or to people who suffer from no illness at all, modern psychiatry has chosen to treat the "unhappiness pool" instead of the "illness pool."[37] The *British Medical Journal* got it right: "a lot of money can be made from healthy people who believe they are sick."[38]

Indeed, half of all psychiatric patients are seen in (more lucrative) private practice, and almost half of all patients in private practices have symptoms that are not debilitating or profound enough to add up to illnesses. A World Health Organization study found that, in the United States, about a third of people in psychiatric treatment either met no criteria for a mental disorder or had subthreshold conditions.[39] As Shorter said in a 2003 article, "So Many Left Out: The Seriously Ill Lose Out to the Zoloft Set": "Your chances of receiving proper care are in inverse proportion to the seriousness of your condition."[40]

Large percentages of people with severe and persistent mental illness are in no care whatsoever. "The majority of those with a diagnosable mental disorder [are] not receiving treatment," wrote the U.S. surgeon general in a 1999 report. Studies published in 1985, 2000, and 2001 found that 50 percent, 42 percent, and 46 percent, respectively, of people with serious mental illness were receiving no treatment for their illnesses.[41] The World Health Organization's massive study on the prevalence of mental illness revealed that in developed countries 35 to 50 percent of people with serious cases had not been treated in the last year, and in poor countries, the figure was 80 percent.[42] A separate study found that of those who received treatment, only 40 percent of people with serious mental illness in the United States were receiving what is considered minimally adequate treatment. And only 15 percent were getting the care they need.[43]

The same tragic imbalance exists in the research world. While people with severe mental illness account for more than half of the direct costs associated with all mental illness, only about a third of NIMH research awards between 1997 to 2002 went to the study of serious mental illness. Furthermore, only 6 percent of all NIMH awards were designated for "clinically relevant" research for people with serious mental illness (research explicitly intended to improve the treatment and quality of care for people with such severe conditions). In giving serious mental illness short shrift, NIMH poured its money into numerous areas of dubious value. While the agency declined reasonable proposals to study bipolar disorder in children, it chose to fund studies of self-esteem in college students. It declined to fund research on postpartum depression but supported work on the hearing processes of crickets. Mental illness is a low priority. In 1999, for each person afflicted by illness, the government spent twelve dollars on cervical cancer for every dollar spent on bipolar disorder. For every dollar spent on schizophrenia, thirty dollars were spent on HIV/AIDS.[44]

Unlike the psychotics, the neurotics pay cash. And the neurotics are significantly less work, too—it's a lot easier to talk in a relaxed fashion with someone about their marital problems, their self-esteem issues, their financial woes than it is to attempt to manage people who think that satellites are shocking them from outer space; who hallucinate about having sex with Jesus Christ; who imagine they are the love child of Sammy Davis Jr. and Kim Novak; who think that their brains are being programmed by the letters and numbers that they see on license plates; who believe that the medications are part of a totalitarian regime to control their minds—all of these true scenarios of people that I worked with—who are constantly going in and out of the hospital and who may be at some risk of killing themselves or others.

By the way, the former is the true fear—media distortions to the contrary. People with severe mental illness are much more likely to hurt themselves, or to be hurt by others, than they are to exert violent attacks on others. A 2005 study showed that more than one-quarter of people with severe mental illness had been victims of a violent crime in the past year—eleven times the rate of the general population.[45] A British study showed that psychiatric patients are six times more likely to be murdered than the average person.[46] Conversely, the violence that the mentally ill perpetrate on others has been enormously exaggerated by the media. A MacArthur Foundation study found that people discharged from psychiatric hospitals were no more violent than their neighbors who were not mentally ill—as long as they did not use substances. It is lack of psychiatric treatment and the use of substances that makes people with mental illness violent. But this is also true of the general population: while people with mental illness and substance abuse problems are five times more likely to become violent than the general population, people with substance abuse problems and no psychiatric problems are three times more likely to be violent.[47]

The primary risk, of course, for the mentally ill is suicide. The rates of suicide for people with severe mental illness are astonishing. About 1 in 10 people with schizophrenia kill themselves.[48] The frequency of suicide in people discharged from psychiatric hospitals ranges from about 20 percent for people who suffer from bipolar disorder to 5 to 10 percent for people with borderline and antisocial personality disorders.[49] Consistent with this research, when I was running facilities I found that what kept me up at night was the fear of my patients hurting themselves and using drugs. I didn't have to worry about my patients hurting other people.

The slippery slope that psychiatry has traversed—jettisoning the impoverished mentally ill for the cash-carrying worried well—can perhaps be traced to a single word choice in DSM-III, the totally revised diagnostic manual of 1980. If not for the selection of that one word, the recent history of psychiatry might be entirely different.

The prevailing term to describe specific psychiatric conditions in the first diagnostic manual, the DSM-I in 1952, was an odd one: *reaction.* Schizophrenia, for example, was described as a "schizophrenic reaction." Depression was a "depressive reaction." The concept of "reaction" derived from psychoanalytic thinking, and as such, mental torment was thought to come about as a result of a reaction to environmental, psychological, and biological problems. By DSM-II, published in 1968, the term *reaction* had been completely tossed aside. DSM-II described depression in more psychological terms, such as *depressive neurosis* and *depressive psychosis.* DSM-III, which was the brainchild of one man, Dr. Robert Spitzer of Columbia University, was an attempt to strike a middle ground between the psychoanalytic camp, which had no interest in biology, and the budding brain scientists, who were starting to gain traction as psychiatric drugs were becoming more prevalent and were often successfully treating people with severe mental illness. Spitzer, who is probably, after Freud, the most influential psychiatrist of the twentieth century, worked on DSM-III for six years, often up to eighty hours a week. In order to appease both groups, Spitzer brought a centrist, "theory-neutral" approach to his work. In other words, he based diagnoses not on theories and traditions about how they might have arisen, but on objective observation and symptoms lists, on "the here and now." While this was no doubt well intentioned, the lack of theoretical constraint meant that just about any painful and unhappy human predicament could be entertained for inclusion.

Spitzer presided over an extraordinary expansion of the DSM. It has been said that Spitzer was "more interested in including mental disorders than in excluding them." "Bob never met a new diagnosis that he didn't at least get interested in," said Allen Frances, a psychiatrist who worked closely with Spitzer on the DSM-III. "Anything, however against his own leanings that might be, was a new thing to play with, a new toy." Spitzer was a technician of diagnosis and loved to compose symptom lists, sometimes drawing them up on the spot.[50] It should be noted that in his centrist approach, Spitzer also presided over many positive developments. For example, he removed homosexuality as a diagnosis, which had been notoriously included in DSM-II. Spitzer also excised "hysterical personality" disorder—which had become unfairly identified with female instability. (The word *hysteria* itself comes from uterus—hence the term *hysterectomy*.)

The word that Spitzer settled on to cover the vast majority of all three hundred diagnoses was *disorder*. *Disorder* had the same bland, theory-neutral qualities. It was not *neurosis* or *reaction* (both heavily associated with psychoanalysis), nor was it *disease* or *illness* (terms associated with the brain scientists). *Disorder* wasn't entirely new: it had appeared briefly in earlier DSMs to describe general categories of distress. Everybody was happy—or, perhaps, everybody was unhappy. The problem is that *disorder*, so bland and toothless, so appeasing to all parties, has little meaning. There are few constraints on the word *disorder*. Just about everything can be a disorder.

Spitzer's word choice, well-intentioned and politically expedient as it was, created the overly broad territory that psychiatry occupies today. Had Spitzer settled on, say, the word *disease* instead, it is conceivable that the whole course of modern psychiatry would have been different. Diseases are scary, upsetting, painful, often chronic, and potentially lethal. You stay in bed with diseases. People don't like to be around you when you have a disease. You generally don't look well when you have a disease. By contrast, having a disorder is, generally speaking, no big deal. It can mean that you're just a "little off," just need a little boost, that you'll probably be okay soon. If you're at a cocktail party and tell someone you have a disease, they might step back. If you tell them you have a disorder, they're likely to ask you questions about it. Do you think that 11 percent of American women would be taking antidepressants if depression were defined robustly as a disease? Do you think a psychiatric journal could argue that nearly 50 percent of the population has met either threshold or subthreshold criteria for a depressive or anxiety disorder, if they were instead called depressive and anxiety *diseases*?[51] Would Americans have flocked by the millions to certain lesser diagnoses, if they had been defined as diseases? It's one thing to say, at the office holiday party, that you have social anxiety disorder; it's quite another to say you have social anxiety disease. Had GlaxoSmithKline been marketing Paxil for generalized anxiety *disease*, it would have been a much harder sell. The ads on prime-time TV would have been much more distasteful.

The use of *disease* as the prevailing term for psychiatry, while in my view a vast improvement, would not always be appropriate. *Disease* can connote contagion, not relevant to psychiatry, and is also associated with viral conditions. If biological psychiatry has taught us anything, it is that the major psychiatric diagnoses are in fact diseases of the brain. As an alternative, the term *illness* could be employed, which it is quite often by experienced clinicians: as in, "depressive illness," "bipolar illness," "schizoaffective illness." But generalized anxiety illness and seasonal affective illness, alas, don't quite have that requisite Madison Avenue ring, either.

It's unlikely that the next version of the DSM will change any terminology. "My sense is that the DSM has become such a moneymaker for the American Psychiatric Association that we shouldn't expect anything terribly revolutionary in the next version," Roger K. Blashfield, a psychology professor at Auburn University who has written a great deal about the politics of psychiatric diagnosis, told me. Indeed, the DSM-IV and the revised edition, DSM-IV-TR, together have sold 1.4

million copies at about eighty dollars apiece,[52] making it one of the more lucrative books in recent publishing history.

So the most recent diagnostic manual of the American Psychiatric Association is happy to provide any number of diagnoses for disorders and issues that are patently not for mental illnesses at all. For practitioners unwilling to slap Julie with major depression, there are any number of alternatives. If Julie was going through a major life change, she could be diagnosed with:

> ADJUSTMENT DISORDER, defined so robustly as: "The development of emotional or behavioral symptoms in response to an identifiable stressor(s) occurring within three months of the onset of the stressor(s). These symptoms or behaviors are clinically significant as evidenced by either of the following: (1) marked distress that is in excess of what would be expected from exposure to the stressor or (2) significant impairment in social or occupational (academic) functioning."

Or, if she was having troubles on the job, with:

> OCCUPATIONAL PROBLEM: "An occupational problem that is not due to a mental disorder or, if it is due to a mental disorder, is sufficiently severe to warrant independent clinical attention. Examples include job dissatisfaction and uncertainty about career choices."

Or, if she was questioning her sexuality, with:

> IDENTITY PROBLEM: "Uncertainty about multiple issues relating to identity such as long-term goals, career choice, friendship patterns, sexual orientation and behavior, moral values, and group loyalties."

Or, if she was getting a divorce, with:

> PHASE OF LIFE PROBLEM: "A problem associated with a particular developmental phase or some other life circumstance that is not due to a mental disorder, or, if it is due to a mental disorder, is sufficiently severe to warrant independent clinical attention. Examples include problems associated with entering school, leaving parental control, starting a new career, and changes involved in marriage, divorce, and retirement."

Or, let's say a recent dispute with her daughter is what is troubling Julie, with:

> PARENT-CHILD RELATIONAL PROBLEMS: "A pattern of interaction between parent and child (e.g., impaired communication, overprotection, inadequate discipline) that is associated with clinically significant impairment in individual or family function or the development of clinically significant symptoms in parent or child."

Or, let's say it's difficulties with her sister, with:

> SIBLING RELATIONAL PROBLEM: "When the focus of clinical attentions is a pattern of interaction among siblings that is associated with clinically significant impairment in individual or family functioning or the development of symptoms in one or more of the siblings."

Or, it's something so vague and diffuse that we don't really know what it is, with:

> RELATIONAL PROBLEM—NOT OTHERWISE SPECIFIED: "Relational problems that are not classifiable by any one of the specific problems listed above (e.g., difficulties with coworkers)."

The psychiatric diagnostic term *Not Otherwise Specified*, or *NOS*, is a wonderful conceit. NOS appears in the DSM "whenever symptoms are so vague, so mild, or so untreatable"[53] that they don't deserve a full-fledged diagnosis. My favorite encounter with the NOS concept occurred when I was working in a supportive housing program for formerly homeless people with mental illness. My client Jamaal was so ill that he had features of many disorders, but not enough to make a clear diagnosis in any one area. He was obsessive, depressed, anxious, *and* psychotic. In preparing my case review, I agonized over Jamaal's proper diagnosis and ended up proposing about ten potential ones. Our team discussed the merits of each one, carefully reviewing the DSM criteria, and attempted to rule them out or in accordingly. We could arrive at no clarity. The supervising psychiatrist, Dr. Moore, a truly wise doctor, sighed and interrupted me. "You know when you were growing up," he said, "there were some kids who were just weird? And then they just got weirder and weirder? That's what I think Jamaal is—he's just weird. He's just a really weird guy. I think he's Weird NOS." From then on, Weird NOS is how I thought of Jamaal.

So this is how slippery the slope has become:

On April 1, 2006 (note the date), *The British Medical Journal* ran a story introducing a new disorder: motivational deficiency disorder, or MoDed. The article went:

> Extreme laziness may have a medical basis, say a group of high-profile Australian scientists, describing a new condition called Motivational Deficiency Disorder. The condition is claimed to affect up to one in five Australians and is characterized by overwhelming and debilitating apathy. Neuroscientists at the University of Newcastle in Australia say that in severe cases motivational deficiency disorder can be fatal, because the condition reduces the motivation to breathe. Neurologist Leth Argos is part of the team that identified the disorder, which can be diagnosed using a combination of positron emission tomography and low scores on a motivation rating scale, previously validated by elite athletes. "This disorder is poorly understood," Professor Argos told the *BMJ*. "It is underdiagnosed and undertreated" . . . A study of the economic impacts of moti-

> vational deficiency disorder estimates the condition may be costing the Australian economy $A2.4bn a year in lost productivity . . . Professor Argos is an advisor to a small Australian biotechnology company, Healthtec, which is currently concluding phase II trials of indolebant, a cannabinoid CB1 receptor antagonist . . . the preliminary results from the company's Phase II trials are promising, according to Professor Argos: "Indolebant is effective and well tolerated. One young man who could not leave his sofa is now working as a financial investment adviser in Sydney . . ."[54]

It turns out that MoDed, as any reasonably intelligent reader would ascertain, was a spoof, created by a group of enterprising journalists and academics—who clearly did not suffer from MoDed—at a conference on "disease mongering." And *The British Medical Journal*, which has a tradition of running humorous pieces in its April 1 issue, went along with it. But the joke was not universally appreciated, apparently; a number of respectable news outlets picked up the news release and published stories of the sensational new disorder "without a hint of skepticism."[55] And so the developers of MoDed proved their point: how gullible our present culture is to the claims of new diseases and their remediation.

Extreme anger is also, apparently, a major mental illnesses. In 2006, *The Archives of General Psychiatry* soberly ran an article called "The Prevalence and Correlates of DSM-IV Intermittent Explosive Disorder in the National Comorbidity Survey Replication." Respected Harvard researchers analyzed World Health Organization data and reported the alarming news that "intermittent explosive disorder" was far more common than previously thought. The disorder, according to the article, is characterized by tirades during which the sufferer destroys property, attempts to hurt or actually does hurt someone, or threatens to do so. Depending on how narrowly it is defined, the prevalence of intermittent explosive disorder ranges from 4 to 7 percent of the population, with a mean of forty-three lifetime attacks resulting in $1,359 in property damages.[56] "We never thought we'd find such high prevalence rates for this condition," said the lead author, Dr. Ronald Kessler, apparently shocked that so many of his countrymen are so . . . well, angry.[57] Shopaholism is also being explored as a bona fide psychiatric ailment. Stanford researchers have been evaluating the use of SSRIs for "compulsive shopping disorder," which they also describe as a hidden epidemic.[58] When I was talking to a colleague in a New Haven coffee shop about the rise of "shopaholism," a fellow diner, overhearing us, asked to speak to me. She confided that she suffered from the disorder and asked me for help.

To which I say: nonsense. Anger, greed, laziness, impulsivity, as well as jealousy, lust, anguish, and so on are simply part of the human predicament. They are not medical conditions. To treat them as medical conditions is a perversion of medicine. This is by no means to minimize the pain and suffering of nonclinical problems. Divorce, poverty, job instability, family feuds, sexual identity questions, and the like can, of course, be extremely painful. But however painful and urgent, these problems of living are not medical problems and are better addressed, as we shall see, by nonmedical interventions: counseling, informal support, social networks, better communication in relationships, as well as exercise, hobbies, and creative self-expression.

In the overdiagnosing spirit of the times, I have suggestions for the forthcoming edition of the DSM. I think we've got to get beyond the absurd vapidity of "Phase of Life Problem" and "Sibling Relational Problem." Let's get a little more specific about Julie's angst. Let's take the daring step of calling life problems what they are, and what they were, up until about twenty years ago: life problems. Here are my modest proposals for Julie's true diagnosis:

Bummed Out Disorder
Scared of the Professor—NOS
How Can I Afford My SUV Disorder
The Doctor Said I Look Depressed, So Why Don't You Take Zoloft? Disorder
Worried That My Son Is Gay Disorder
My Husband Is Not There for Me Disorder

Loneliness Disorder
I Don't Like to Speak in Public Disorder
Weird, Unsettling Feelings of Anxiety That Come and Go Disorder.

Lest you think my suggestions too flip, let me assure you they are real. Years ago I worked in a university department with a group of women. They were as normal as pie. In time, as I got to know them, the majority of them revealed to me that they were taking, or had recently taken, SSRIs. Having administered hundreds of SCIDs—the Structured Clinical Interview for the DSM-IV—as a psychiatric researcher, I can testify that none of them have had major depression or an anxiety disorder or a panic disorder or a body dysmorphic disorder. These were eminently sane women going through some rocky times. The above list accurately describes what was actually troubling them. Ultimately, all of them got off the medications, whether in a few months or a few years. One said that the meds made her agitated and crazy; one said they didn't do much for her, except calm her down at times and make her fat; and one said she didn't quite know why she was taking them, but they did numb her out sufficiently to get her through some hard times on the job.

For the moment, I would like to toss aside the DSM and its half-baked fatuous terminology.

Here's my diagnosis for the untold millions of Julies: Miserable—Not Otherwise Specified

Admittedly, this may not be a clinical and certainly not a reimbursable diagnosis, but there is ample evidence that over the last two decades numerous forces have been causing Americans to be ever more isolated, under pressure, and emotionally entitled. In short, miserable. This is a new kind of American misery—there have been others: civil wars, world wars, economic depressions, recessions, malaise. But current forces are creating a new kind of "misery index," beyond the fiscal one invented by the Yale Economist Arthur Okun in the 1970s: Economic Misery Index = Unemployment Rate + Inflation Rate.

Here's my take on the new Misery Index:

Emotional Misery Index = Isolation + Pressures to Be Happy + Pressure to Turn Inward

I would contend that it is the forces of isolation and pressure to be happy and pressure to turn inward and not any truly diagnostically valid form of depression that are driving the vast majority of Julies to look at themselves in the mirror in the middle of the night, wonder when things are going to get better, and reach for their Prozac. This is a distinctly contemporary kind of disenchantment and disappointment. The great short story writer John Cheever put it in a slightly different way: "The main emotion of the adult American who has had all the advantages of wealth, education, and culture is disappointment."

Isolation is of course a critical factor. Social connectedness is highly correlated with well-being; conversely, isolation is highly correlated with rates of mental illness and distress.[59] Isolation causes depression, and depression causes isolation. The aforementioned Martin Seligman, characterizing depression as a disorder of "*individual* helplessness" (italics are mine), believes that rampant individualism, and the isolation associated with it, is perhaps the leading cause of the epidemic of depression. "In the past, when we failed, as fail we must, there was spiritual furniture to fall back on for consolation. Our relationship to God, our patriotism, extended families, community . . . Systematically, in the two generations in which depression has increased so drastically, we've seen waning of all these spiritual furnitures."[60] How important is social connectedness? Roughly speaking, if you belong to no social groups but then decide to join one, you cut your risk of dying in the next year by roughly half.[61]

But by virtually every social measure, according to such comprehensive and masterly studies as Robert Putnam's *Bowling Alone: The Collapse and Revival of American Community*, Americans are increasingly living in their own atomized and self-absorbed realities. Even as the lives of most Americans have become more materially comfortable and technologically more convenient, our Edward Hopperish aspects—the isolated brooding, solitary existence of people passing each other at late-night diners—have become ever more pronounced. Even as communication technologies have proliferated and become vastly more sophisticated, we have become ever more incommunicado, living in our own comfy but sterile and increasingly virtual private spaces, accessed through TV and computer screens, which indeed screen out much of the irksome nature of much of the world. More and more, we choose to live in our own "Private Idahos"—a phrase popularized by the 1981 hit song with the refrain "You're living in your own Private Idaho."

The dominant image of the era is the American driving alone to work in his massive and luxuriously equipped climate-controlled SUV, unaware even of the road beneath him, talking on his cell phone or listening to one of a hundred satellite radio channels. The Lonely American stares into a computer screen all day long, writing reports, writing e-mails, trading stocks half a world away, and then returns to the glorious SUV bubble to ride to a home that's not on a real street but in an artificially created enclave (homogenous "planned residential development," or gated community, or "high-end" condo) and into his automated garage, leading to his 3,000-square-foot McMansion, and then watches one of three hundred satellite channels or surfs one of three billion sites on the Web, until bedtime, all to repeat the next day. The McMansion might provide solace, except that it is double mortgaged and the home improvements and high-tech accessories are financed by maxed-out home equity lines. Lately, cocooning has taken on a new wrinkle—the creation of and deep immersion in our own customized on-demand "digital environments," which combine the realms of Web surfing, video games, instant messaging, cell phones and their photographic and text messaging capabilities, cable TV, DVDs, and on-demand television and movies. Vincent Bruzzese, the author of a study that showed that young males had attended 24 percent fewer movies in the summer of 2005 than in the summer of 2003, said, "The digital environment has really captured the hearts and minds of everyone, and particularly younger males. They are staying home at an incredible rate right now."[62] As my sister-in-law said, "Not even the kids play outside anymore."

Many of the popular TV shows present unending torment and misery. They are either "reality" shows in which gorgeous contestants eat live locusts while hanging provocatively from airplanes with their cleavage showing, or truly brutal crime dramas, featuring decapitations or the sexual molestation of children or the murder of bystanders. The reality shows, of course, are not reality at all, but the most curiously manufactured and contrived settings: let's bring ten unrelated and very attractive people out to a private island, create false scenarios of danger, and give the winner a million dollars. The purpose of all this appears to be solely to distract viewers from the mundane features of their own lives and let them feel better about their own dissatisfactions. As in: their lives life may be difficult and drab, but at least live scorpions are not at their feet. The crime shows have becoming vastly more technical and "forensic" in their presentation. Crimes are re-created in slow-motion, frame-by-frame detail, ballistics experts are called in, semen samples are tested for DNA—all creating an ever more voyeuristic and gruesome level of detail, all in deceptive service of the plot. In fact, there is less and less actual plot, and more and more of the various forms of torture.

Ours apparently not being a comedic age, there are few sitcoms anymore, and the only breakthrough domestic drama of recent years has been the appropriately named *Desperate Housewives*, in which one of the housewives gets addicted to her child's Ritalin. There aren't new crime shows, either, just spin-offs from preexisting franchises, like fast-food restaurants: among the most popular TV shows are *Law and Order*, *Law and Order: Special Victims Unit*, *Law and Order: Criminal Intent*, *CSI*, *CSI: Miami*, and *CSI: New York*. The Lonely American's one nod towards any participation or even awareness of a larger, communal, national life is the placement of a yellow ribbon decal, in honor of the troops in Iraq, on the SUV's bumper, or a bumper sticker that makes some general statement about "freedom" and "liberty." Otherwise, he is curiously buffered from the pressing causes of the day—save for his bumper sticker, it's as if a war doesn't exist, and no one seems to care or notice that, for example, the rich keep getting richer and the poor poorer.

The second component of the new misery index is the pressure to be happy. What underlies this is an entirely new phenomenon in American history, a novel sense of what I call "emotional entitlement." By emotional entitlement, I mean a very recent but endemic belief on the part of vast swaths of Americans that we should feel happy all the time, or at least most of the time, and that the conditions of life/society/the very existence of drugs/fill in the blank should allow us, as much as possible, to maximize our feelings of happiness. In some ill-defined but nonetheless pervasive way, we have come to feel we are entitled to—*no, we are owed*—happiness. This is a wholly new creation in the mental landscapes of America: first introduced in the 1960s and 1970s, when the pursuit of individual bliss first became possible and supportable; then reinforced in the 1980s, with its renewed emphasis on individual gain; and finally confirmed in the 1990s and 2000s, when entitlement, in the sense of being owed something you haven't necessarily earned, became a widespread American attitude.

The SSRIs are at the epicenter of emotional entitlement, its ultimate symbol and its ultimate expression. Whether or not one has actually taken SSRIs, their mass existence has served to reinforce the widespread notion that one *should* be happy, and if one is not, there is a mechanism available to make one so. This expectation, of course, has nothing to do with the actual efficacy of the pills themselves. In this sense the impact of the SSRI revolution may be more symbolic than actual. The enduring legacy of the Serotonin Empire may not be the pills themselves but their allegorical value. Like nothing else before in American history, the SSRIs instilled in the public the idea—entirely independent of the clinical utility of the pills—that there exists something "out there" that can make them happy. The implications of this fundamentally wrong belief have been profound and largely destructive.

The growth in America of entitlement to material things has spilled over into immaterial things. In *The Good Life and Its Discontents*, Robert J. Samuelson traces the origins of the contemporary uses of the term *entitlement*, which he defines as "specific government programs, in which benefits are promised if people (or institutions) meet explicit legal standards." (He may as well have added "whether they really need them or not.") According to Samuelson, by that definition, *entitlement* first appeared in a long-forgotten 1944 law. It then disappeared from political and popular discourse for decades. It resurfaced only in the early 1980s. In 1981, *US News & World Report* identified what the magazine deemed a "revolution" in entitlements; and the term appeared in *Time* and *Business Week* later that same year. Reagan was the first president to use the term commonly—one can surmise in what context.[63]

Not long ago, Americans didn't feel entitled to anything at all. There simply wasn't much to be entitled to. As Samuelson points out, it is startling to take inventory of the things that didn't exist in America before World War II. As recently as 1940, there was virtually no government safety net. Health insurance was uncommon, and pensions barely existed.[64] Most people rented, and most houses were heated by wood and coal. More than half of households lacked a refrigerator and about a third didn't have running water. Nearly half the labor force worked in farm, factory, mining, or construction jobs.[65] Should one be unable to support oneself and one's family, there were few alternatives other than the poorhouse, the state hospital, or religious and charitable organizations, and the taint or moral shame associated with those institutions was profound and extreme. It's only recently that supports of various kinds have been in place. While Social Security was established in 1935, it didn't become a major feature of American life until well after World War II. In 1945, only half a million people received Social Security benefits;[66] Medicaid and Medicare weren't created until 1965. Both of those programs also got off to relatively slow starts but now are massive components of the federal budget. Persons served by Medicare mushroomed from 7 million in 1967 to 27 million in 2002.[67] Collectively, the entitlement programs of Social Security ($488 billion), Medicaid ($300 billion), and Medicare ($176 billion) now make up almost half of the federal budget.

Feeling entitled to all this, we think we are also entitled to happiness. Although the United States was founded on the credo that "We hold these truths to be self-evident, that all men are created equal, that they are endowed by their Creator with certain unalienable Rights, that among these are Life, Liberty and the pursuit of Happiness," it's only recently in human history, in the years preceding the Declaration of Independence, that happiness has even been on the agenda. Thomas Carlyle observed in 1843, " 'Happiness our being's end and aim' is at bottom, if we will count well, not yet two centuries old in the world." Before the seventeenth century, "happiness," in our modern sense, pleasure or good feeling, was a morally and spiritually dubious pursuit. For most people, existence was truly Hobbesian—nasty, brutish, and short. Only in the last century or two has there been a softening and relenting of the notion that life is unending misery and sin and that suffering is actually good and ennobling: the more one suffers, or tolls, or sacrifices, the more virtuous one is, and the closer one will get to heaven. It is also only relatively recently in the course of history that the individual sense of self—as an autonomous entity free to pursue its own desires and whims—has emerged. And even then, Thomas Jefferson, in crafting the Declaration of Independence, did not mean happiness in our modern, follow-your-bliss understanding of the word. "Our greatest happiness . . . is always the result of a good conscience, good health, occupation, and freedom in all just pursuits," he wrote. What drove the pursuit of happiness was classical as much as Christian. Jefferson was well versed in the classics, and he took from Aristotle and Cicero the notion that happiness "was the final end of human existence, the goal of a life well-lived." This, writes Darrin M. McMahon, author of *Happiness: A History*, "was happiness attained through discipline, self-sacrifice and reasoned moderation." "Happiness is the aim of life," Jefferson affirmed, "but virtue is the foundation of happiness." To Jefferson, virtue meant serving others and working to enhance the public good. Virtue transcended the selfish interests of the individual. The way to ensure "the happiness and freedom of all," he stated in his first inaugural address, was to perform "all the good in my power."[68]

But we surely take happiness seriously now. Various indicators from the whimsical to the putatively profound indicate that happiness has become a serious business. From the omnipresence of that uniquely

American icon, the smiley face, to the prevalence of emoticons (the smiley faces of e-mail discourse), to Web sites like myspace.com that allow the user to register their mood at every entry, to the birth of a burgeoning new academic field, Happiness Studies, with its own journal, the appropriately named *Journal of Happiness Studies*, it is clear that happiness is something that Americans feel terribly compelled to pursue.

Perhaps the final critical factors in the new misery index are the forces that have pushed us inward, to contemplate only ourselves. I submit that at the heart of this inward turning is the evolution of that uniquely American concept, psychological and physical, of the Frontier.

It would seem that, until fairly recently, America has always had the Frontier. From the early English settlers on, there have always been two constants in the American domain—"the pale" (i.e., civilization, or some version of it), and "beyond the pale," the line beyond civilization (where the Indians were, or in later iterations, where the Mexicans, the Cubans, the Russians, the Sandinistas, the Grenadian rebels, the Palestinians, the Ayatollah, bin Laden, al Qaeda, and the Iraqi insurgents were, or are). Writing in the late nineteenth century, the visionary historian Frederick Jackson Turner believed that it was the notion of the Frontier—specifically, the wrestling with and conquering of the Frontier—that made America into itself:

> Thus American development has exhibited not merely an advance along a single line but a return to primitive conditions on a continually advancing frontier line, and a new development for that area. American social development has been continually beginning over again on the frontier. This perennial rebirth, this fluidity of American life, this expansion westward with its new opportunities, its continuous touch with the simplicity of primitive society, furnish the forces dominating American character.[69]

Turner believed that taming the frontier uniquely imbued our culture with self-reliance, or as he phrased it, "the frontier is productive of individualism." Turner attributed all American "exceptionalism" to the frontier: the "coarseness and strength combined with acuteness and inquisitiveness," "that masterful grasp of material things," the "restless, nervous energy," "that practical, inventive turn of mind, quick to find expedients," and the "freshness, and confidence, and scorn of older society, impatience of its restraints and its ideas, and indifference to its lessons."

I submit that the existence of the Frontier, or lack of it, has enormous psychological implications. For example, the relative lack of a formidable physical frontier in Britain (resulting from the relatively small size and scale of the country) has surely contributed to the prominent and abiding role of restless imagination and exploration in that culture. It broke one of two ways—inward or outward—depending on the temperament of the explorer. Inward-looking souls were drawn to the imagination and created intricate inner worlds. Why do the best children's authors—Lewis Carroll, C. S. Lewis, J. M. Barrie, J. K. Rowling—come from Britain? Why did Shelley write *Ozymandias*? Because their authors, bored with or having exhausted the extent of their physical surrounds, were compelled to invent their own imaginary frontiers. For outward-looking, physically adventurous types, the lack of a frontier on native soil meant that they had to go looking for one in all corners of the globe. The British became the greatest explorers, navigators, governors, and exploiting rulers in the world. They produced the British Empire. And when the empire effectively closed, there was a resulting depression and turning inward in postwar British society. Walker Percy commented that since the empire went dark, the British, once the global elite, have been the world's best practitioners in only three areas: spying, the writing of mysteries and detective novels, and acting. All of these trades share a duplicity with, and a remove from, the surfaces of reality. Once the limits of the physical world were explored, and then lost, there was no place for British talent to go but inward.

The problem in America is that the Frontier is now closed. Writing in 1893, Frederick Jackson Turner had already pronounced it so. He declared at the end of his famous essay: "And now, four centuries from the discovery of America, at the end of a hundred years of life under the

Constitution, the Frontier has gone, and with its going has closed the first period of American history." Turner was seventy-five years premature in his declaration. There were many, many worlds left for Americans to conquer, or at least fight or sometimes just defend, in the upcoming century—Europe during the world wars, communism, the global economic marketplace, the global cultural marketplace . . .

Perhaps it is possible to identify the exact moment that the American Frontier was symbolically closed—at just about ten in the evening on July 20, 1969, when Neil Armstrong walked on the moon. That moment of transcendence—"one small step for man, one giant leap for mankind"—was also the moment at which we had pushed the physical world to the maximum. Americans had explored our available world to its outer reaches. "Beyond the pale" ceased to exist. There have, of course, since that time been multiple other attempts at space exploration and at pushing the American empire's boundaries in skirmishes across the globe, but many have failed and none have extended the frontier farther than Neil Armstrong did. (Alternatively, one could argue that the door to the Frontier was finally slammed shut with the January 28, 1986, explosion of the Space Shuttle *Challenger* that killed all seven astronauts on board.) Somewhere in the last few decades, American forward movement has gotten stuck. No longer is there any attainable final frontier, other than the imaginary one on *Star Trek*.

With nowhere stunning and glorious left to go, Americans are now left only to explore their own psyches, their own inner journeys. After Neil Armstrong's triumphant stroll, the place to go has been inward. There's nowhere to go but to the Self-Help aisle, to *I'm Okay, You're Okay*, to Hare Krishna, to Transcendental Meditation, to Scientology, to twice-weekly psychotherapy, to Alcoholics Anonymous, AlAnon, Narcotics Anonymous, Overeaters Anonymous, to biofeedback, to bulimia and anorexia, to generalized anxiety disorder, to social anxiety disorder, to sibling-relational problem—not otherwise specified, to chemical imbalances, to Zoloft and Prozac and Paxil, and to Julie with her depression with a small *d*. We have ended up not on the moon but isolated and feeling that we need to be happy, while on hold with the managed-care company, listening to Muzak and trying to get information from a customer service agency in India about the coverage of antidepressants.

Fortunately, as shall be explored in the second half of this account, there are alternatives. It is possible to do better. The second half of this book will propose different ways of looking at the problems of depression and anxiety and even suffering itself. Specifically, cognitive-behavioral therapy, which has been shown repeatedly to be an effective form of treatment for depression without drugs, will be explored. I will also investigate important new nondrug approaches to engage patients into treatment and motivate them to change.

It is important to stress that many of the ideas covered in the coming chapters are little known outside the field of psychiatry and even within the mainstream parts of the field. The reason for that is simple. What follows are ideas, not products. There is no money to be made off of them, and hence, they have not been commodified into the larger culture. There are no marketing budgets, no product detailers, no prime-time DTC commercials, and certainly no fortunes to be made from these approaches. That virtually no attention has been lavished upon them does not mean they cannot be meaningful and life changing. And in the place of hype, there is data that shows they can help many people.

What there is is research data that shows they can be effective for many people. There are also a few caveats to keep in mind. All the modest proposals that I will explore are extended in the spirit of offering help and solace and improvements in symptoms and functioning. But none, it should be made clear from the very start, offer a permanent end to depression and anxiety, to trouble. The treatment of mental torment is a murky and complicated business, and no panaceas exist. It is the belief that such a cure-all agent exists that has created the massiveness of the psychiatric drug industry in the first place.

The other caveat is that the approaches explored in the coming chapters require earnest work and a strong commitment to get better. These treatments and approaches require action instead of passivity—

the patient can no longer just be a vassal—a mere recipient of a pill—but must take the lead and be in charge of their own treatment and their own recovery. This requires, unfortunately, sweat and bother.

All of which is to say that the suggestions to come are not as simple and easy as taking a pill, hoping for the best, and not calling the doctor in the morning. But countless lives have been improved and even saved through these alternatives and drug-free approaches.

PART TWO

A Series of Alternative Approaches

CHAPTER FIVE

Cogito, Ergo Sum

Perhaps psychoanalysis and Aaron Beck were just never really meant for each other. You see, he had a happy childhood. "I grew up with loving parents, which was a problem when I was in psychoanalysis. I could not recall any unpleasant experiences in growing up."[1]

Nonetheless, as a young psychiatrist in the 1950s, Aaron Beck trained to become an orthodox analyst (at the famed psychoanalytic center Austin Riggs, where he studied with Erik Erikson, and at the Philadelphia Psychoanalytic Institute). And early in his career, he was quite enthusiastic about the potential for psychoanalysis to improve the world. "I was a strong believer during and after my psychoanalysis that this approach was for everyone, and I tried to persuade my friends to become analyzed."

There was a specific moment that changed everything. It came when Beck, freshly graduated from analytic training, was treating a provocative young woman. She lay on the couch relating one lurid story after another about her sexual adventures with men. Beck scrupulously took notes.

Beck asked her, "How does talking about all this make you feel?"

"Anxious," she said.

Beck responded as a well-trained analyst should and attempted to probe the deep inner conflicts that lay under the evident symptoms.

"You are anxious," the young doctor declared, "because you are having to confront some of your sexual desires. And you are anxious because you expect me to be disapproving of these desires."

"Actually, Dr. Beck, I'm afraid that I'm boring you," the patient replied.

It turned out that the patient wasn't obsessed with hidden sexual conflicts and early childhood experiences with her father. As Beck continued to ask her exactly what she was thinking in the moment, it became clear that the patient was involved in a constant, suffocating inner dialogue that told her she was worthless, unattractive—and boring. All of which she was not. It turned out that her promiscuity was rooted in her wanting something to offer men in order to compensate for her supposed inadequacies.

From that time on, Beck started asking his patients very simply what was going through their minds in the present moment, in the here and now. This was not what one was supposed to do as a psychoanalyst. But it opened up a whole new world, a direct and transparent view into the psyche.

In this encounter with the young woman, the seed of what was to become cognitive-behavioral therapy (CBT) was born. It would take Aaron Beck another twenty years to fully formulate, test, and refine his cognitive techniques. But now CBT is the most empirically validated psychotherapy in the world—about four hundred outcome trials have shown its efficacy for a broad range of psychiatric disorders, as well as for medical disorders with psychological components.[2]

The trick is absolute directness. One of the "cardinal" questions of CBT, according to Judy Beck, Aaron's daughter, who now runs the Beck Institute for Cognitive Therapy and Research in suburban Philadelphia, is simply: "What was just going through your mind?" By posing that simple question, Aaron Beck discovered that his patients were plagued by what he eventually called "automatic thoughts." Automatic thoughts are those words and images that fly through our minds, usually rapid-fire, while we are talking or reacting or waking up or walking down the street. We all have them constantly—and Beck discovered, in plumbing the automatic thoughts of his patients, that he himself had them all the time without really being aware of them.

Beck found that for depressed people, automatic thoughts were at the core of their problems. They clog up the works and lead to a series of distortions. Automatic thoughts are not considered and evaluated in the way other thoughts are; they are simply believed to be true, and then we flit ahead to the next one. In depressed people, automatic thoughts are particularly distorted. Over years of study and work with patients, Beck found that the automatic thoughts of depressed people are marked by a pervasively negative view of themselves, the world, and the future. Furthermore, there was a "straight line" between the thoughts and mood. A situation would occur, it would provoke negative automatic thoughts, and that in turn would lead to a depressed, ugly mood. The basic idea behind CBT is that thinking controls or largely affects behavior. If you change thinking, you have a good chance of changing behavior. As Alfred Adler, a psychotherapist who developed a precursor to CBT, stated, "I am convinced that a person's behavior springs from his ideas." CBT is actually based on a very old idea in Western culture, specifically the work of the Stoic philosophers, including Epictetus and Marcus Aurelius. Epictetus wrote in *The Enchiridion*, "Men are disturbed not by things, but by the view which they take of them."

In experiments, Beck found that after a successful or positive experience, "depressed patients had a positive shift in mood, increased optimism, and increased motivation."[3] Creating such a positive feedback loop for patients disconfirmed their negative feelings about themselves. With these findings, Beck started CBT by focusing on practical methods to increase patients' objectivity regarding their feelings about situations and encouraging them to take an active role in "cognitive restructuring": replacing the automatic thoughts with more realistic appraisals of the situation and their place in it. Many of his patients would get better in five or ten sessions, a stark contrast to the open-ended, often years-long format of psychoanalysis. For the first time in history, Beck proved the efficacy of a form of psychotherapy for depression.

"I started off believing that I was going to practice psychoanalysis for the rest of my life, but when I started observing patients' automatic thoughts, I thought it much better to have them sit up [off the couch] so that I could look at their expression and nonverbal communication. I would ask them what was going through their mind at the time . . . When I focused on these negative thoughts, patients began to get better fairly soon. Patients whom I thought would be with me for a year or two or three reported, 'I am finished, Dr. Beck; you have helped me a lot and I do not need you anymore.' My clinical load shrunk enormously."

Over time, Beck codified a number of specific types of thinking errors:

All-or-nothing thinking. This involves viewing situations in only two extreme categories instead of along a continuum. Example: "If I'm not a total success, I'm a failure."

Catastrophizing. The tendency to predict the future negatively without considering less extreme, more likely outcomes. Example: "I'll be so upset, I won't be able to function at all."

Disqualifying or discounting the positives. Unreasonably telling oneself that positive experiences don't matter. "I did that project well, but that doesn't mean I was good at it. I just got lucky."

Emotional reasoning. Thinking that something must be true simply because one feels it. "I feel like she's mad at me, so she is." "I know I do a lot of things pretty well at work, but I still feel like I'm a failure."

Personalization. Believing that others are behaving negatively because of you, without taking into account more likely explanations. "The repairman was mean to me because I did something wrong."

Overgeneralization. Sweeping negative conclusions that go beyond the specific situation. "Because I felt uncomfortable at the meeting, I don't have what it takes to make friends." "Because I stuttered twice at the job interview, there's no way they're going to hire me."

Mind reading. The belief that you know what others are thinking. "He's thinking that I don't know the first thing about this project." "I know she thinks I'm a fool."

Should *and* must *statements, or "imperatives."* Having a fixed idea of how one should behave and overestimating the consequences when those expectations are not met. "It's terrible I made a mistake. I must always do my best."[4]

As he burrowed deeper, Beck found that automatic thoughts were based on what he called core and intermediate beliefs, many of them emanating from childhood or critical experiences that form basic notions of our identity. Examples of core beliefs would be "I'm the rebel," "I'm the peacekeeper in the family," "I'm the smart one," "I'm the unreliable one," "I'm the protector." Intermediate beliefs are slightly more specific. For example, from the "I'm unreliable" core belief, the intermediate belief would be "I can't manage money." Beck also identified how behavioral and physiological reactions arise from automatic thoughts.

The following is an example of the cognitive model adapted from Judith S. Beck.[5]

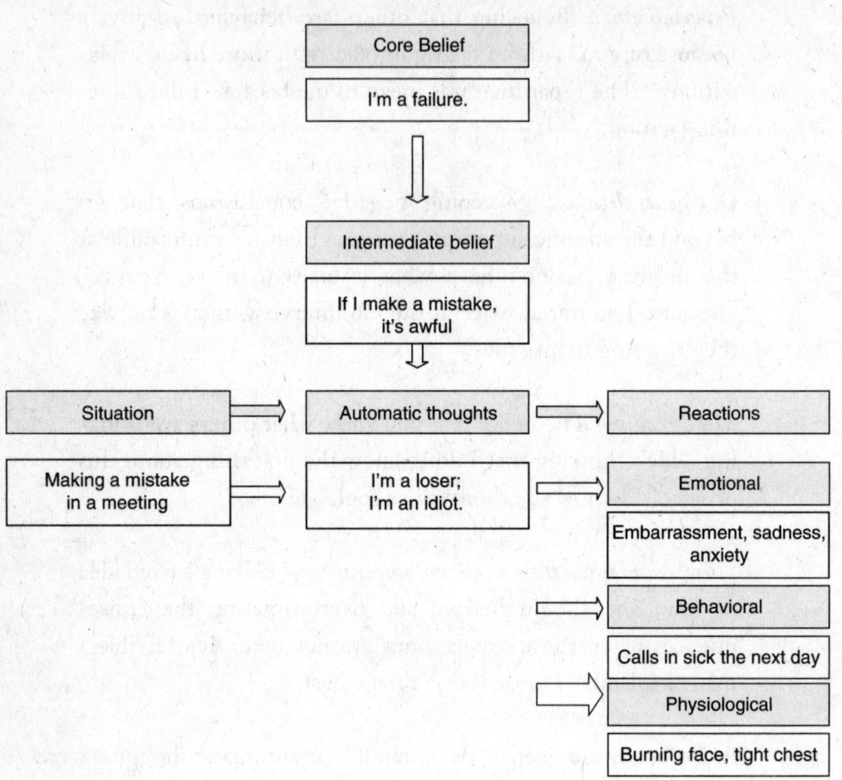

Beck and others eventually merged newly discovered behavioral techniques, arising from the work of B. F. Skinner, into CBT. (A note on terminology: the Becks like to call their therapy, rooted as it is in the cognitive model of their own devising, simply *cognitive therapy.* But as cognitive therapy adapted behavioral techniques, the name *cognitive-behavioral therapy* emerged. The more inclusive *cognitive-behavioral therapy* is now the term most widely used in psychology and psychiatry.) Behavioral tools include relaxation exercises, increasing activities that give the person a sense of pleasure or accomplishment, and exposure and desensitization exercises, whereby the person will over time expose themselves to a triggering situation, in order to gain control over it and reduce the anxiety and fear associated with the trigger. For example, if a person had a phobia (phobia reduction is a tremendously efficacious application of CBT) of crowds, the therapist would first have the person think of going to a crowded place, then have the person actually go near or pass through a crowded place, and finally have the person stay in a crowded place for a period of time. This process would be guided by the therapist, and the client would report back on their progress at each session. In most cases, with repeated exposure, the client learns to respond less negatively to the offending stimulus.

Aaron Beck also formulated some basic principles for CBT. An essential one is the creation of "a sound therapeutic alliance" between therapist and patient, one of collaboration. Therapist and patient operate under the transparent assumption that they are working collaboratively to identify and solve the patient's problems. While such a principle might seem obvious, there have been plenty of therapies that have not been based on a collaborative relationship. Some therapies have used confrontational approaches, or, in order to create "the blank slate" upon which the patient can freely project their dreams and fantasies and so on, the therapeutic hierarchy has been made necessarily unequal.

So nakedly collaborative is CBT that the therapist is instructed to ask for feedback from the patient at the end of each session. "What was helpful?" "Was there anything I didn't understand?" "Is there anything you'd like to do differently next session?" CBT is also formidably goal-oriented. Usually, the patient's goals for treatment are identified at the beginning of the first session, and progress toward those goals is evaluated weekly. CBT is also time-limited, usually twelve to fifteen sessions. The intent is that by the end of the treatment the patient will have learned the cognitive-behavioral, and problem-solving skills so that they can do the work on their own.

In 1975, Beck founded the Center for Cognitive Therapy at the University of Pennsylvania, where he treated thousands of patients and trained a new generation of doctors. In 1994, he founded the nonprofit

Beck Institute for Cognitive Therapy and Research, now run by his daughter. Aaron is in his eighties and is still going strong. In recent years, he has been evaluating CBT for schizophrenia and for the prevention of suicidal behavior, among other psychiatric disorders.

Beck ultimately came to the conclusion that psychoanalysis was a "faith-based therapy." Armed with now hundreds of studies, Beck can claim CBT as an empirical therapy. My personal view of psychoanalysis is that just because it is essentially devoid of a research basis does not mean that is not useful for some people. When analysis suits the right learning and personality styles of its recipients (and it is best suited for patients who are verbal, insight-oriented, and already motivated for treatment—admittedly a small subset of the psychiatric population), it can be enriching and meaningful.

Of course, there was the inevitable and obligatory fallout from the analysts. Upset by his defection from the camp, analysts informed Beck that the problem must have been that he "had not been well analyzed."[6]

Aaron and Judith Beck are rather like their therapy: eminently straightforward, the ultimate straight shooters. Unlike Freud, who took cocaine, and the Freud disciple Karen Horney, who slept with patients, or Carl Jung, who was off in the clouds, or B. F. Skinner, who shocked rats and wrote utopian novels that seemed also somehow cruel, or Albert Ellis (another early discoverer of cognitive approaches), who was reckless and combative, Beck comes across as the Boy Scout of therapists. He loved the Boy Scouts. "The greatest learning experience I ever had probably was as a Boy Scout. I had to learn things that were quite difficult for me—lifesaving, swimming half a mile . . . I think that if there was any pattern in my life it was going out and meeting challenges that lay before me. I think I was conscious of that and I would galvanize myself. I had a strong need to conquer whatever problems I faced."[7]

Aaron comes across as a Norman Rockwell–style pediatrician, complete with bow ties. He has four children and eight grandchildren. His wife is a superior court judge. Aaron grew up as the third son of Russian Jewish immigrants in Providence, Rhode Island. He almost died at age eight, from a staph infection that developed after surgery for a broken arm. Two of his siblings died in childhood. His father was a socialist and a printer who wrote poetry. His mother likely suffered from depression. Beck attended Brown University and Yale Medical School. Two of his children, Judith and son Daniel, are cognitive therapists. A third son, Roy, is a neuroopthamologist and epidemiologist.

I asked Judith Beck if she has used CBT on herself.

"Of course," she said without hesitation or embarrassment.

"Can you give me an example?"

"I have a son, with some special needs. When he was younger, he suffered from a terrible seizure disorder, sometimes suffering up to a hundred seizures a day. I would get quite anxious, and I catastrophized that as an adult he would never be able to leave home, that he would be socially isolated, that he would never be able to work, and that he would be unhappy. And then, in a systematic way, I would attempt to decatastrophize those thoughts and replace them with more realistic scenarios. I would repeatedly rehearse and summon up an image of him, as a young adult—of him being cared for, of being able to work, of being basically okay. That was a major thing for me. It helped me get through a hard time."

"And how is he doing now?"

"Quite well. During the midst of all those seizures, his doctor put him on a Ketogenic diet.* Would you believe that his seizures went down to one or two a year? He's attending a special post–high school program. He's really doing okay."

Dr. Lisa Fenton is a pleasant, clear-eyed, sharp-looking woman, perhaps in her late forties. Her office is in a twenty-story apartment building on the farthest reaches of the medical school campus. There aren't many twenty-story apartment buildings in New Haven—or in Connecticut, for that matter—and, if not for the expansive, quiet, and rather tired-looking park outside her window, it would seem that we were somehow in the middle of Manhattan.

Lisa's office, along with other Yale behavioral health offices, is

*A high-fat, low-carbohydrate diet used to control seizures.

located up and down the corridor of the second floor. ("Behavioral health" is the latest politically correct name for the field of mental health—the thinking being that *mental* is too narrow a term to encompass all the realms of emotion and action and that it has connotations of "mental hospitals" and "mental illness." While the intention is no doubt noble, I find the term *behavioral health* also to be limited. The problems are not limited to behavior; any phrase to describe what Lisa Fenton and other therapists do has to include a reference to feeling and thinking, to inner states.) That Lisa's office is in an off-campus apartment building is a reflection of overcrowding at the medical school, so that peripheral enterprises like behavioral health get spilled out onto the margins. But I believe the setting, perhaps unintentionally, makes a statement: this is treatment offered and rendered in the "community," away from the confines—literal and figurative—of the hospital and its clinics and inpatient units.

She didn't intend to become a cognitive therapist. She was "psychodynamically" trained—meaning psychotherapies that draw on psychoanalytic theory to help people understand the roots of emotional distress—but when a grant at Yale came along that required a cognitive therapist, she decided to get training. She went to Philadelphia and was trained at the Beck Institute by Judith Beck and others.

Lisa describes one of her patients.

"Martha came to me. She was thirty-five, and she was married, with three children, one with severe special needs. Another child was an infant. I saw her weekly for three months, and now I see her once a month for just a few more sessions. She came from a very high-functioning family that wanted her to be a lawyer. She merely became an accountant, and that bothered her family. Her husband was an illustrator, and his employment went up and down. At the time Martha came to me, he was not working, and they were under financial pressure. When I first saw her, she was quite depressed. She couldn't sit still, she was so agitated. She had quit her job because she felt so disorganized. She was cognitively scattered, hopeless, and despondent. She told me that she was actively suicidal. She was thinking about it all the time and had even looked into her life insurance policy to see what the payment would be if she died, and if it covered suicide.

"She'd had suicidal ideation—constant thoughts of suicide—even as a kid. She'd had one previous really serious bout of depression when she was in college. At that time she took Prozac and then stopped it after two or three months. This depression was much more severe. She came to me saying that she wanted to try treatment again but without medications.

"When we began to examine her reactions to situations—her automatic thoughts—and what lay beneath them, it turned out she had a core belief that she was damaged, a defective person, that would kick in whenever a difficult situation occurred. Let's say her husband, tired, came home from work and was upset that the house was a mess. And how could it not be sometimes, with an infant and a child with special needs. Let's say he complained about it. Martha would immediately go to: 'I'm a failure as a wife. He doesn't love me. He's going to leave me.' And that would very quickly go to thoughts of suicide. And even plans of suicide. She was also highly perfectionistic and would despair when things weren't the way they were supposed to be—like having a messy house, which is of course a totally normal situation when you have young children!

"So a lot of our early work was spent on reevaluating that core belief and replacing the cognitions that flowed from it with more realistic ones. So we spent quite a lot of time—it came up in parts of just about every session—talking about the very hypercritical atmosphere in her house growing up, the fierce expectations of her parents, and how as a result, she believed that she was somehow not up to the task, was indeed inferior and damaged. We spent some time looking at how that negative and faulty belief about herself affected how she perceived whole parts of her life. When she made a mistake at work, or wasn't able to keep things quite in order at home, the negative belief would get triggered and result in increased feelings of depression. The only solution that seemed to make sense was suicide. When she was able to formulate a more realistic view of herself as a mostly competent but human individual, she was able to better tolerate the natural imperfection in her life. We would go through those automatic thoughts and work on replacing them with more realistic ones. So to the thought that her husband is going to leave her, I would say, Is there any evidence for that? Has he ever left you before? No, she would say, he has never even talked of splitting up. I would ask: Is there any evidence that he does love you? And she would say: He told me that he loved me yesterday, and he's told me he thinks I'm a good mother, and he supports me coming to this therapy, and so on. Ultimately, she was able to identify that the suicidal ideation was based on faulty thinking.

"I would give Martha homework assignments to do between sessions. She would write down the Core Belief, the Intermediate Belief, the Situation, the Automatic Thought that arose, and the Feelings and Reactions that came out of that. Then she would test those automatic thoughts, and we would work over time on replacing those cognitions. Also, at the start of every session, she completed a depression inventory, a twenty-one-question form, to probe the severity of depression. At the beginning, her score was twenty-two: solidly in the moderate range of a major clinical depression. We started to see those scores go down. She would complete that form by herself at the beginning of each session, bring it to me, and then we would review it together. We would work on lowering her perfectionistic standards from 100 percent perfect to maybe 80 percent perfect.

"We didn't have to do too much work on behavioral engagement, like increasing the number of pleasurable activities in her life. When she started looking at her thinking, she was able to start to do some things again. She started taking a writing class, which is something she always wanted to do.

"Our therapy is winding down. Martha is now considering a career change, something more creative where she can use writing. Some kind of link between the business world and writing.

"By the end, she started looking better. She was always attractive, never unkempt, but she looked like she was dressed up to look good last time I saw her. She appears a lot less overwhelmed and perplexed about things. She is not at all tangential, and she is not jumpy like she was.

"Last time I saw her, we had missed the previous few weeks because of holidays and the like. She told me that she missed me but that she didn't feel dependent on me. That's when I knew things were working. It was not so much that I had been so great—like it wasn't about me—but that she had learned the skills on her own."

"And what was her last score on the depression inventory?" I ask.

Lisa goes to look through the chart.

"Four," she says. "That's subclinical."

No doubt Dr. Fenton chose a particularly winning example of a CBT treatment for me to hear. (Although there was little preparation in her response; I merely asked her to tell a treatment story, and she told this one without much forethought.) Later, what most impresses me is this: as part of the grant under which she works, she and her psychiatrist collaborator are required to refer their patients for a medication consult if their depression scores do not go down significantly over the course of the treatment. The men and women Dr. Fenton treats are severely depressed, and often under great stress, and sometimes under extreme financial hardship. (Because it is part of the research grant, the treatment is free.)

"How often do patients ask for medications?" I ask.

Lisa has to think for a moment. "Not all that often," she says. "About a third do. That doesn't mean they didn't improve with the CBT, though."

CBT sometimes has a "bad rap" in psychiatry for lacking imagination, for being tied to a script or a manual, for not being sufficiently free or creative. I am struck in talking to Lisa that she does not use a manual. "I just stick to the core principles," she says. "For each patient, I deploy them differently. So, for example, with Martha, we did spend a great deal of time in the early sessions on the formulation of her core belief of being defective, because that was so pronounced and so clearly tied to the expectations of her family. And then we didn't have to spend much time on behavioral matters, because she was able quickly to reengage with pleasurable activities in the world. For other patients, it might be just the opposite. This is what keeps it interesting—it's different with every patient I work with."

Similarly, Judith Beck says she uses self-disclosure with most patients. "Self-disclosure often gives them [the patients] a different way of thinking about their problems," she says. "And it goes a long way in strengthening our relationship when patients recognize that I am a human being who is willing to share something of herself to help them."[8] This practice would be anathema to traditional psychotherapy! Judy also says that a skilled therapist also needs to be able to target different types of thoughts and beliefs, depending on the disorder. For depression, it is typically negative thoughts about the self, the world, and the future. For phobia, it's the catastrophizing and misinterpreting of thoughts and beliefs that cause the symptoms. For obsessive-compulsive disorders, it is not so much ideas about the self that cause the problems, but about the object of their obsessions. And so on.

Cognitive-behavioral therapy has been shown to be "as effective and possibly more effective" than drugs in managing mild to moderate depression.[9] For people suffering from moderate to even severe depression, CBT can be as effective as medications.[10] For insomnia, CBT has been shown to be more helpful than the sleep aid Ambien. In 2004, CBT was shown to help alleviate hypochondria in six sessions and, in conjunction with drugs, to help depressed adolescents and kids with obsessive-compulsive disorder. There are currently about 150 clinical trials being conducted to test CBT for an ever-widening number of problems: Tourette's syndrome, gambling addiction, obesity, irritable bowel syndrome, and as a therapy for sexually abused kids.[11]

It also has no side effects—unless you count the homework. (This is meant as a joke, but not really—the fact is that CBT requires real effort, focus, and resolve.) But the main difference between CBT and drugs lies in the relapse rates: that is, the return for a duration of at least two weeks of the symptoms of a significant depressive episode. A review of eight studies that compared remission rates of depression for people who were treated either by CBT or by medications showed that 30 percent of people treated with CBT relapsed with depression, compared with 60 percent of those treated with antidepressants.[12] Furthermore, analyses from some studies have also shown that the dropout rates from treatments with CBT are significantly lower than those from treatments with medication.[13] Altogether, CBT has been shown in several studies to be more cost-effective than medications.[14]

Even for severe conditions like bipolar disorder, for which medication is absolutely appropriate, the addition of CBT to a medication regimen makes a great difference. Patients were rehospitalized at significantly lower rates and had better ratings on mood, social functioning, and coping.[15]

These are important findings, and they make an eminent amount of sense. With the comprehensive approach of CBT, you are actually going to the root of the problem and providing patients with skills that they can deploy repeatedly over time to marshal against triggers and remissions. It involves a lot more than the numbing of symptoms. "We believe that cognitive therapy might have more lasting effects because it equips patients with the tools they need to learn how to manage their problems and emotions," said Robert DeRubeis, professor and chair of the University of Pennsylvania's Department of Psychology and author of one of the studies. "Pharmaceuticals, while effective, offer no long-term cure for the symptoms of depression."[16] Jonathan Abramawitz, a psychologist at the Mayo Clinic, has said of cognitive therapy, "It's like learning to ride a bike. You are practicing these skills over and over. No one can take them away from you for the rest of your life. The long-term benefits of cognitive therapy are better than medicine because with medicine, when you stop, the symptoms come back."[17]

To pick an example of CBT's potentially life-changing effectiveness: people who had recently attempted suicide and who received ten sessions of CBT were 50 percent less likely to try to kill themselves again than those who did not receive the therapy. The CBT groups attempted to help find a more effective way for patients to deal with problems, such as managing negative thoughts and feelings of hopelessness. Patients examined the thoughts, feelings, and actions that lay behind their previous attempts and worked on strategies to respond differently to stress in the future. These promising results have tremendous public health implications. "Since even one previous attempt multiplies suicide risk by 38 to 40 times, and suicide is the fourth leading cause of death for adults, a proven way to prevent repeat attempts has important public health implications," said the Director of the National Institute of Mental Health, Thomas Insel.[18]

CBT has some highly practical applications. Researchers in the physiotherapy department at King's College, London, administered a cognitive-behavioral pain management program for patients experiencing chronic pain after cancer treatments such as surgery, radiotherapy, and chemotherapy. A group of patients, most of whom had suffered from breast cancer, were taught cognitive and relaxation techniques and exercise training. They met with a therapist only an average of ten times. The results, published in the lyrically entitled *Journal of Pain*, showed that those who underwent the CBT pain management training had improved rates in coping with pain, increased fitness, and lower rates of anxiety and depression.[19]

Cognitive-behavioral treatment is significantly associated with reducing criminal behavior, unlike psychotherapy, which has been shown to increase it. (Unstructured psychotherapy has been proven to be disastrous for certain groups, such as criminals, making them more likely to recommit crimes. As a colleague of mine quipped, "They may be more likely to re-offend, but at least they have a better understanding of why they do it.") A substantial body of scientific research has consistently found that participants in cognitive-behavioral programs have recidivism rates that are 10 percent to 30 percent lower than rates for offenders who did not receive such services. Among the general population of prisoners, cognitive-behavioral treatment has decreased recidivism by about a third. Larger gains have consistently been noted with higher-risk prisoners.[20] Cognitive-behavioral treatment programs for prisoners have been shown to be dramatically cost-effective. Studies have estimated that there are financial returns of between two and eleven dollars for every program dollar invested in cognitive-behavioral treatment, while punishment-oriented programs have cost the system money, resulting in returns of only fifty to seventy-five cents for every dollar spent.[21]

So as it turns out, Tony Soprano probably would have been better served by CBT than by Prozac. As Tony lamented to Dr. Melfi after a year of Prozac: "Medication, medication, medication! What do I got to show for it?"[22] (Actually, at one point Dr. Melfi is about to refer Tony to CBT and get him off her hands, but she changes her mind.) Tony suffers from antisocial personality disorder—for which, most mental health professionals would say, there is not much effective treatment—and panic disorder, for which CBT is absolutely indicated. But the screenwriters of *The Sopranos,* even if they knew a lot about CBT, would not have written much of it into many episodes. Prozac, and Tony's conflicts with his mother, make for a better script.

In the high-tech age of Corporate Psychiatry, efforts like CBT don't get the press they should. As Lewis Opler, medical director of the New York State Office of Mental Health, told me, "Cognitive-behavioral approaches are underutilized in this country."[23] As are even simpler interventions, like diet and exercise. Evidence is accumulating that basic lifestyle choices have a huge impact on depression. Fish oil, for example, appears to be very good stuff for the brain and behavior, which makes sense because omega-3 fatty acids have a critical role in brain development and functioning, including promoting the growth of neurons in the frontal cortex. Fish oil has been shown in a series of studies by Andrew Stoll at Harvard to ease the symptoms of bipolar disorder and depression. This line of research was provoked by the observation that in countries where a lot of fish is eaten, like Japan, depression tends to be low. Omega-3s cannot be made by the brain and need to come from diet, mainly seafood. Mothers in England who consumed little fish during pregnancy experienced dramatically higher rates of postpartum depression than women who ate fish regularly.[24] Bernard Gesch, of the University of Oxford, enrolled prisoners in a study of diet. Half of the prisoners got a placebo; the other half got a diet rich with vitamins and fish like salmon. For the inmates with the better diet, the assaults and other disciplinary violations went down by a third, over time. In a similar trial concerning people with a history of substance abuse, symptoms of "anger" on the part of the group with better diet were reduced by half.[25]

Exercise also is undeniably an effective treatment for depression, even for major depression. Many studies have shown this. Researchers at Duke University found that the reduction of symptoms was similar for those who received Zoloft alone, undertook 30 minutes of exercise three times a week, or both.[26] In addition, as in the case of CBT, those in the exercise conditions had significantly lower relapse rates at ten months.[27]

Glen Gabbard, of the Baylor College of Medicine in Houston, has compiled a comprehensive literature review on the effectiveness of psychotherapy, described in part below. Dr. Gabbard is a particularly interesting and broad-minded psychiatrist who has written variously and convincingly about psychoanalysis, the convergence of neurobiology and psychotherapy, and the treatment of personality disorders, as well as writing a popular book, *The Psychology of* The Sopranos: *Love, Death, Desire, and Betrayal in America's Favorite Gangster Family*.

It turns out that psychotherapy, which nobody has paid all that much attention to in the neuro era, and which has suddenly seemed old-fashioned and low-tech, if not downright wimpy compared to our fascination with million-dollar brain-imaging machines and chattering neurotransmitters, has consistently been delivering impressive treatment outcomes across a range of human predicaments. Psychotherapy has lost so much ground in recent years that longtime staples of therapy-influenced conversation have all but disappeared. When was the last time someone accused you of a Freudian slip? When was the last time someone wanted to analyze your dreams? All that has been replaced by talk of chemical imbalances and hardwiring. But unglamorous as it has become, accused at times of being merely an expensive form of hand-holding, the fact remains that psychotherapy helps people feel and function better. A broad analysis of many studies found that by the end of psychotherapy, the average treated patient is better off and functioning better than 80 percent of untreated patients.[28] Family therapy reduces the relapse rate in patients with schizophrenia to the same degree—50 percent—as antipsychotic medications.[29] For children with anxiety and depressive disorders, intensive psychoanalytic treatment at four to five times per week was more efficacious than therapy one to three times per week. Also, the longer the duration of the treatment, the better the outcome.[30]

In general, social support, whatever its form, is critical to healing. Sheldon Cohen, a psychologist at Carnegie Mellon University, says: "The most striking finding on relationships and physical health is that socially integrated people—those who are married, have close family and friends, belong to social and religious groups, and participate widely in those networks—recover more quickly from disease and live longer. Roughly eighteen studies show a strong connection between social connectivity and mortality."[31] Cohen would know. He has studied risk factors of the common cold and has found that stressful personal relationships make a person significantly more likely to get a cold. Bad relationships are as much a causal factor for the common cold as vitamin C deficiency and poor sleep.[32]

There is also a convincing literature that psychotherapy, which managed-care companies in their penny-pinching myopia have been so loathe to pay for, saves a lot of money in the long run. It has been repeatedly substantiated that the proactive and preventive nature of psychotherapy reduces the usage of far more acute and expensive services, such as emergency room visits and hospitalizations. A review of the English-language literature on psychotherapy over a ten-year period, from 1984 to 1994, found that in almost 90 percent of studies, psychotherapy for patients with severe psychiatric and substance abuse disorders produced cost savings by reducing hospitalizations, medical expenses, and work disability.[33]

When the United States military expanded psychotherapy coverage for dependents, a savings of $200 million over three years was generated from reductions in psychiatric hospitalization. For each dollar spent on psychotherapy, four dollars were saved on more intensive services.[34] Twice-weekly psychotherapy with borderline personality disorder patients (which any experienced clinician will tell you is a notoriously difficult condition to treat and manage) over a yearlong period decreased higher-cost use of psychiatric inpatient services, emergency room care, and appointments with other medical specialists. The work performance of patients also improved. Savings were calculated at $10,000 per patient per year.[35] A study of psychotherapy and psychoanalytic patients in Germany found that treatment decreased medical visits by one-third, lost work days by two-fifths, and hospital stays by two-thirds. The longer the treatment lasted, the more successful the outcome.[36]

In addition, in recent years, ironically coinciding with the Corporate Psychiatry era that began in 1988, psychotherapy has improved a great deal. The techniques of psychotherapy and the understanding of effective psychosocial approaches have become much more sophisticated. The one-size-fits-all approach of long-term, fairly unstructured, verbally oriented psychoanalysis or dynamic psychotherapy has been replaced by a number of new approaches specifically geared towards the needs and styles of the patient. Psychoanalysis and psychotherapy absolutely work well for verbally minded "worried well" people, with a fair degree of insight about their problems and motivation to do something about them. But it clearly doesn't work for other people. The "recovered memories" of early life abuse and trauma uncovered by psychotherapy have proved to be highly unreliable and have often resulted in the retraumatization of the patient. What works better for victims of such trauma is a very direct, specific approach—based not on mining the past, but focused on improving the present. Short-term crisis counseling immediately after a traumatic event—the kind practiced by no doubt well-intentioned social workers and psychologists who descend on dazed victims and witnesses after some immense tragedy, like school shootings and Hurricane Katrina and 9/11—has been shown to be unhelpful, and sometimes destructive.[37]

Medication or therapy, it is important to understand that there are no panaceas. One must understand and accept that there are no magic bullets, no cure-all agents to rescue us from oblivion. In the realms of psychiatry and mental health, there are no penicillins (nor, I posit, will there ever be) to stop illness and disease in its tracks. It is the hope and belief that such a magic bullet or intervention exists that got us into trouble with all this overmedication in the first place. As successful as it is, CBT is no elixir. To say that it helps 60 percent of patients, for example, is to say that it doesn't work for 40 percent of them. (This is not at all unusual in the discipline of medicine generally. Despite ongoing medical progress, there seems to be an enduring Rule of Thirds across most treatments: a third get better, a third stay the same, and a third get worse.) Emory University psychologist Drew Westen, who has treated what he calls "refugees" of cognitive therapy that didn't work out, has found that many patients have benefited from his longer-term approach. Westen feels there is now a "a tremendous bias" toward CBT in psychiatry.[38] And sometimes the depression can just be too strong for CBT. "I've seen people who have done hard work in cognitive therapy, but they just can't sustain it when depression returns," says Jerrold Rosenbaum of Massachusetts General Hospital.[39]

The other problem is that CBT has not entered the mainstream culture, nor may it ever. Psychoanalysis, while devoid of much research base, was a lot of fun. It was the stuff of dreams, stories, conflicts, sex, aggression, unconscious desires, Freudian slips. It even offered a couch to lie down on! CBT, perhaps to its detriment as an art if not a science, is not narrative- or interpretation-based.[40] CBT is a highly effective carpentry of the soul, therapy as technology or engineering as compared to art. This is to its credit as a science but not as a product to be marketed.

But there are signs it may be taking hold. Twice as many psychologists follow CBT as psychoanalytic or psychodynamic approaches. Over half the cases at Integrated Behavioral Health, which manages the mental health benefits for companies employing 1.5 million Americans, now involve a provision for CBT, up from 10 or 20 percent a decade ago.[41] There is a new requirement that all psychiatric residency programs teach CBT.[42] CBT was the subject of a cover article in *Forbes*—of all places—in 2006. Judith Beck's 2007 diet book, *The Beck*

Diet Solution, despite being turned down by major publishers, became a surprise best seller. The book offers a cognitive approach to dieting. "I counsel people to learn a different cognitive or behavioral skill each day for two weeks before they even start a diet," she told me. "The big publishers all wanted immediate solutions, and they all wanted me to include a specific diet in the book. That's not what it's about. I'm interested in the long-term approach of changing our thoughts and beliefs toward food. The behaviors, and the specific diet, all that comes later." The week that I interviewed her, she appeared on *Good Morning America*.

And most significantly, in 2006, Aaron Beck won the Albert Lasker Clinical Medical Research Award. The Laskers have been called America's Nobel Prize, or the pre–Nobel Prize. Since 1967, no fewer than seventy-one Lasker honorees have gone on to win the Nobel Prize, most within two years of receiving the Lasker. Aaron Beck was the first scientist working in the area of psychotherapy to be so honored.

The British government and National Health Service are considering making a major investment in CBT. Lord Layard, a Labour peer and a former advisor to the prime minister, has proposed that the National Health Service invest £600 million to train and hire 10,000 CBT therapists, who would work in a network of 250 psychological centers across the country. Characterizing mental illness as "our biggest social problem," Lord Layard hopes that through his initiative a million people would be treated by CBT.[43] Layard had the ear of Tony Blair, after the former prime minister became convinced of its medical, social, and economic benefits.[44] CBT was even part of the Labour party platform in 2005.[45]

Another intriguing aspect to cognitive-behavioral therapy, and one that may also contribute to its popular breakthrough, is its curious but undeniable connection to the "mindfulness" of Eastern approaches, Buddhism in particular. CBT has been characterized as Buddhist in spirit in the manner in which it stays in the here and now and increasingly, practices acceptance. It has been observed that Buddhism can be viewed as a psychology as well as a religion, and that Buddha was in fact the first psychologist. Buddhism—2,500 years old compared to CBT's fifty—is based on the Four Noble Truths: (1) life is full of suffering; (2) the root cause of suffering is attachment to worldly things and worldly ideas; (3) it is possible to cease suffering, based on the extinction of and detachment from one's attachments; and (4) the pathway out of suffering is to follow the Eightfold Noble Path, which includes mindfulness and concentration. In its preoccupation with suffering and its relief, Buddhism has a natural resonance with mental health and psychiatry.[46] "If we can reorient our thoughts and emotions, and reorder our behavior, not only can we learn to cope with suffering more easily, but we can prevent a great deal of it from starting in the first place," wrote His Holiness the 14th Dalai Lama, in an uncanny summary of cognitive principles.[47]

Marsha Linehan, a psychologist at the University of Washington, has been the most explicit articulator of the connections between CBT and Eastern approaches. Linehan was formally trained in cognitive-behavioral techniques, which she applied to the condition of borderline personality disorder. Borderline personality disorder is perhaps the most notorious of psychiatric diagnoses. People who suffer from borderline personality disorder tend to engage in stormy interpersonal relationships, in which other people are regarded in seemingly capricious and extreme terms: back and forth from wonderful or horrible, exalted or devalued. People suffering from this disorder appear to lack a stable ego identity. Lady Diana almost certainly had a borderline personality disorder, and Marilyn Monroe probably did. The Glenn Close character in *Fatal Attraction* was a borderline par excellence.[48] (I am not being misogynist in citing female examples. The disorder is far more common in women, particularly young women.)

For a long time, borderline personality disorder was essentially thought to be untreatable. It was largely believed that all a therapist could do with a severe borderline was attempt to set limits and be as consistent and firm and composed as possible, which is of course very difficult to do. To this day, many psychiatrists refuse to treat borderline patients. Experienced therapists know what can lie ahead—the 3:00

a.m. calls to the beeper, the demands to be seen on a Sunday, the histrionics and drama. The stories are legion of Upper East and West Side psychiatrists wisely dropping off their patients at the hospital for the month of August before they went on vacation on the shores of Cape Cod. Yet about one in ten people with borderline personality kill themselves, and while they often are capable of meting out a great deal of suffering to others, they are in a huge amount of distress themselves. Borderlines account for 20 percent of all psychiatric hospitalizations.[49] Between 40 percent and 70 percent have been sexually abused.[50]

Linehan used CBT techniques with some modest effectiveness, but she found something was missing. That thing was acceptance. So intense and so intractable was the condition that merely working on changing cognitions and behaviors was not enough. Acceptance was needed on two fronts—by therapists, to come to terms with the volatility and storms associated with their patients in order to continue to treat them, and by the patients, to mindfully accept their torments in order to stay with the treatment. Linehan had been trained in a contemplative Christian tradition called "centering prayer" and was intrigued by Zen Buddhist principles. In 1985, Linehan took a sabbatical in which spent three months studying with a female Zen master at California's Shasta Abbey and another three months with a Catholic priest also trained in Zen. "It was utterly clear to me afterwards that I had found what the patients needed," Linehan says. "I just had to figure out how to teach it to them."[51] But she knew that patients would not have the capacity to meditate for hours, and many of them had little religious tradition to draw upon. Linehan needed to "take the Zen out of Zen." Linehan developed a new therapy, Dialectical Behavioral Therapy, a blend of behavior therapy and "acceptance-based treatments." The *dialectic* in DBT refers to the contrast between changing feelings and behaviors and accepting them.

Among the core skills that Linehan proposed was that of mindfulness, which involves enhancing the patient's ability to observe, describe, and participate. *Observing* here is developing the capacity to watch events in more appropriate ways, rather than either recklessly plunging into or abruptly abandoning a relationship or situation, which many people with borderline personality disorder have made careers of. *Describing* is "the ability to apply verbal labels to behavioral and environmental events" that are "essential for both communication and self-control."[52] In other words, being able to delineate the differences between the inner and outer worlds, which can be very difficult for borderlines. *Participating* in this sense is entering completely into the activities of the current moment and learning to focus the mind and awareness on the current moment's activity, rather than splitting attention among several activities, or between a current activity and thoughts about something else. All of it has to do with living in the here and now, and more rationally assessing and operating in the moment. "You'd be amazed at how much suffering is due to thinking about the future or ruminating about the past." Linehan has said.[53]

Linehan is a veritable star in the mental health world. Hers is one of the few names that engender almost universal respect in the contentious and polarized world of psychiatry. Her Dialectical Behavior Therapy books and manuals have sold hundreds of thousands of copies and are de rigueur on any contemporary psychologist's bookshelf. Patients who participate in DBT have fewer hospitalizations, healthier social adjustment, fewer suicidal gestures, and drop out less from treatment.[54] This is not to say that DBT is a cure-all for borderline personality disorder. It is merely the best thing yet found to slow down this terribly painful condition.

I have seen DBT work. Around the time Linehan's work was being widely disseminated, I worked with a young woman in Connecticut who suffered from depression, bulimia, and borderline personality disorder. She had gone to Wellesley and dropped out after her freshman year. She was then hospitalized for two years. She was sexually impulsive, volatile, and prone to cutting herself. (She was also charming and brilliant and a hard worker.) She was in a DBT group and she took to it naturally, applying herself assiduously to the workbooks and the homework. She learned to self-regulate her emotions much more tolerably for her (and for the rest of the world). One time I came to her apartment right after she had cut herself. There was blood everywhere. She immediately began to do relaxation exercises and other exercises that are also part of the Linehan curriculum. A week later, she was able to successfully analyze with me what she had done, explain why (her reason at the time was "to feel something"), and identify thoughts and feelings to replace the desire to cut herself. Over time, the self-destructive behavior diminished, and she returned to school, transferring to an Ivy League university. She loved the work of Marsha Linehan. When she read the DBT books and used the workbooks, it was like she was collaborating directly with Linehan in order to get better.

For her part, Linehan is happy. "I always said that in my life I'd go to hell and get people out, and I think I've done that."[55]

Even Aaron Beck has gotten into the Buddhist act. Or perhaps the Dalai Lama has gotten into the cognitive-behavioral act. The Dalai Lama (who has a strong interest in psychology and neuroscience) and Aaron Beck held a public dialogue at the International Congress of Cognitive Psychotherapy in Sweden in 2005. There is a delightful picture of Dr. Beck and the Dalai Lama on stage, clutching hands and beaming. Beck in his bow tie, the Dalai Lama in his gold and maroon robes, holding a public dialogue about the similarities between Buddhism and CBT.

Afterward, Beck posted on the University of Pennsylvania Web site some thoughts about the encounter and about the crossover between cognitive therapy and Buddhism. This is an edited version:

> From my readings and discussions with His Holiness and other Buddhists, I am struck with the notion that Buddhism is the philosophy and psychology closest to cognitive therapy and vice versa.
>
> . . . Acceptance and compassion were key similarities. Also, in both systems, we try to help people with their overattachment to material things and symbols (of success, etc., something we call "addiction").
>
> He appeared to echo what is also the essence of the cogni-

tive approach, namely self-responsibility rather than depending on some external force to inspire ethical standards.

Below is a list of similarities that I suggested to the Dalai Lama in our private meeting.

SIMILARITIES BETWEEN COGNITIVE THERAPY AND BUDDHISM

I. *Goals:* Serenity, Peace of Mind, Relief of Suffering

II. *Values:*

(1) Importance of Acceptance, Compassion, Knowledge, Understanding."

. . . .

(4) Science vs. Superstition

(5) Self-responsibility

III. *Causes of Distress:*

(1) Egocentric biases leading to excessive or inappropriate anger, envy, cravings, etc. (the "toxins") and false beliefs ("delusions").

(2) Underlying self-defeating beliefs that reinforce biases.

(3) Attaching negative *meanings* to events.

IV. *Methods:*

(1) Focus on the *Immediate* (here and now)

(2) Targeting the biased thinking through (a) Introspection, (b) Reflectiveness, (c) Perspective-taking, (d) Identification of "toxic" beliefs, (e) Distancing, (f) Constructive experiences, (g) Nurturing "positive beliefs."

(3) *Use of Imagery*

. . . .

(5) Mindfulness training.

. . . both systems use the mind to understand and cure the mind.[56]

Perhaps a merger of CBT and Zen will give it the requisite amount of contemporary sexiness to make a major cultural breakthrough. Or maybe simply CBT's outcomes will. To anyone who has walked in depression's dark wood and found something that has made them better, there is reason to cry out the message from the rooftops.

Based on sheer clinical efficacy, there should be no reason why the first part of this book shouldn't have been called Cognitive-Behavioral Therapy, Incorporated. One can only imagine the marketing spree the big drug companies would go on if they were to come across a pill with similar proven efficacy to, say, cognitive-behavioral therapy. Pfizer, Lilly, et al. would unleash a blizzard of commercials on the airwaves. A drug that halves suicide attempts! A drug that reduces criminal recidivism by a third! A drug that cures people of phobias! We would never hear the end of it.

The problem is there's no money in it. Psychologists, social workers, and researchers tend not to be the best marketers in the world. You can get some CBT manuals free of charge, on the Web sites of the National Institute of Corrections. Aaron Beck has said, "The drug companies spend several billion dollars a year on their consumer ads and promotions to professionals. This has created an aura of success" for drugs. "It is difficult to compete with such a juggernaut, but gradually it is becoming apparent that human problems are best solved by human solutions."[57]

The other reason why CBT and other psychotherapeutic approaches are not appreciated as they should be is that they require sheer hard work. The provision of human therapies, unlike drugs, takes time, focus, and real effort. Running a cognitive-behavioral therapy group, for example, as I have done for criminal offenders, takes intensive training and organizational planning. One has to get people to show up on time. Not everybody is motivated. You may have someone who is a toxic presence in the group who brings down morale. To measure treatment fidelity, groups should be audiotaped or videotaped, and a neutral, trained observer should evaluate the materials for adherence to the treatment model. Some people are not comfortable with being taped, and it requires special releases. It's all terribly time consuming and occasionally awkward. It can be messy and difficult. The temptation is to give someone a pill and let them go on their way.

I have another theory why psychotherapeutic approaches work. For all the sophisticated techniques employed, for all the proof that they change the brain in the same way that drugs do, the critical factor may still be that they involve the human touch. This is a delicate thing and still not quantifiable, nor may it ever be. There is something in our constitution that requires the presence of others to make *change* authentic. We are sufficiently insecure that changes in our inner life have to be confirmed in the presence of others, by social experience. The presence of a therapist is critical as, among other things, "a confirmer of reality." This is why we need rituals and graduations; they do not create reality, but they corroborate it. They shore up and make real the changes that have transpired within us. When you interview people after they have gone through a successful CBT group, they're more likely to cite the rewards of the weekly contact and fellowship with others—the fact that others care about them—than they are to speak about newly healthy and positive cognitions and beliefs. The process of change is simply more alive when it is experienced in the presence of another person.

But enthralled as they are with technology, Americans don't get excited about such things. It's far sexier to say my doctor just put me on Prozac than to say my doctor told me to take fish oil and exercise more, and gave me a referral to see a cognitive-behavioral therapist.

CHAPTER SIX

The Human Factor

Besides better therapies, there have been, since the birth of Prozac, a series of new understandings about how to engage people in the process of changing their behaviors and what constitutes true recovery from mental illness. Many of these insights have turned old-school medical dogma upside down. All the traditional notions that the doctor is in charge; that the patient does what they're told; that change occurs along a straightforward linear continuum; that people have to be motivated at the beginning of treatment to engage successfully in it; that recovery from mental illness is independent of the social context and is defined only by the successful remediation of symptoms: all these things have been turned on their heads in recent years. As a result of the work of a number of theorists and researchers, the old tenets have been replaced, one by one, in recent years by the following notions: that change is a complex and nonlinear process; that ambivalence to change and lack of motivation is a normal feeling; that empathy on the part of the therapist makes a huge difference in people's ability to recover; that confrontation and authoritarian relationships between caregiver and client are typically not helpful; that recovery from an illness can exist even with ongoing symptoms. Recovery may actually mean learning how to lead a meaningful life even amid the pain of illness.

At the heart of the sea change are two inextricably related models, the Stages of Change model and Motivational Interviewing. Efforts at engaging people in treatment are especially critical for psychiatric disorders and substance abuse because of the "lack of insight"—the missing awareness that one has the problems that one has, or has any problems at all—that is so prevalent in these conditions. It has been argued that lack of insight is one of the very symptoms of schizophrenia. The waning of motivation and activity is of course also a hallmark of depression. Anything that can be done to raise awareness and engagement in treatment of psychiatric disorders is therefore crucial. After all, even if we had the best possible medications and treatments, they would be useless if people were not sufficiently motivated to embrace them. ("You can lead a horse to water . . .")

When I was first exposed to the Stages of Change model, the experience was like the proverbial light going on. I was working in my first year as a case manager at an agency providing supportive housing for the homeless mentally ill. I was working, or attempting to work, with people suffering from rampant substance abuse problems in addition to their mental illness. For a brief ignorant period, my agency had a zero-tolerance approach to relapse with substances, and we were discharging clients hurriedly and thoughtlessly for their "noncompliance." Though I tried not to, I couldn't stop my moral judgment of my clients' failings, their weakness in the face of temptation. I hadn't had much experience with people with severe addictions, and as with the distinction between Depression and depression, there is no comparison between the hard-core addict and the functioning person who drinks or drugs too much. Armed only with outrage, I found myself increasingly at a loss about what do with my clients, who were doing such things as selling the entirety of their possessions in order to get high. There are certain rote recommendations that I was aware of: tell them to go to Alcoholics Anonymous and Narcotics Anonymous, to go to "90 in 90" (ninety meetings in ninety days), to stay away from the "people, places, and things" that might trigger the desire to use drugs or alcohol—but other than these simple directives, I felt completely stumped. I had no tools with which to work.

What I learned at the training gave me a framework to better understand my patients and their reluctance to change. The Stages of Change model was created by Carlo DiClemente when he was working on his psychology dissertation at the University of Rhode Island with advisor James Prochaska. Prochaska's area of interest was how people change in different types of psychotherapies, and DiClemente was interested in "operationalizing" some broader way of looking at the change process. DiClemente had had a lot of prior experience with people and their struggles: before becoming a psychologist, he had been a priest. When I interviewed DiClemente he told me that he had been trying to give up smoking during the time he came up with the Stages of Change model. Certainly his own personal struggle may have helped inform the direction of his thinking.[1]

The Stages of Change model looks like this:[2]

Stages of Change Model

The model illustrates that for any attempted change, one goes through a series of steps: first, Precontemplation, followed by Contemplation, Preparation, Action, Maintenance, and finally either Termination or Relapse.

Precontemplation is probably where most people are in any process of change. It means they are not considering any change at all. Furthermore, they may not be aware that they have a problem. Addicts who do not think they have a drug or alcohol problem are the classic precontemplators. *Contemplation* is the stage at which people have some creeping awareness that they have a problem and are considering doing something about it. They may be concerned about a behavior, but they are ambivalent about changing it. *Preparation* is when a person sees that the perceived advantage of changing outweighs the consequences of maintaining the behavior. The person is specifically planning changes. They are setting goals, and they may be experimenting with ways to change. They plan to act in the next month. In the *Action* stage, a person is making drastic changes to their habits and lifestyle, and they continue to do this over a three- to six-month period. The Action stage has been described as the honeymoon period, the heady early days of change. Often there are greater challenges ahead. *Maintenance* involves sustaining change and prevention of recurrences. It is the period of prolonged behavioral changes, from six months up to five years. The person vigilantly looks out for and guards against triggers for relapse. *Termination* occurs only after years of successful change. The opposite of exit is *Relapse*. Relapse is the event that triggers the individual's return to earlier stages of change, but a relapser can cycle quickly through the early stages.

This model, as simple as it is, was a radical departure for three reasons. First of all, it conceived change as a dynamic and cyclical process. In the West at least, we are more accustomed to seeing progress and development over time as a strictly linear process. But life is more complicated than that; we are constantly going around in circles and back again. In fact, even the Stages of Change is too sequential; in reality, we dance around all of the above stages in all manner of different sequences.

Second, the model conceives of relapse as a realistic part of the change process. The research shows that most people do not immediately sustain the new changes they are attempting to make, and a return to the problematic behavior is typically the rule rather than the exception. Most people who abuse substances, for example, will need to go through several cycles of the Stages of Change to achieve a lasting recovery.[3] Relapse should not be considered a failure and need not become a disastrous or prolonged occurrence. Furthermore, a relapse does not necessarily mean that a client is no longer committed to change. The moral taint of failure is thereby removed.

The third new element, and for many practitioners this is the critical one (it was for me), is the understanding that one must enlist different strategies depending on where the client is in the Stages of Change. Interventions must be targeted specifically to Precontemplators, Contemplators, and so on, and the approach one takes with individuals at different stages of the process is entirely different. If interventions are not matched to the stages of change, they will likely fail.

Case in point: the classic intervention for people who are abusing or dependent on alcohol and drugs, as I learned, is to instruct them to "go to a meeting," to encourage attendance at AA and NA. It is assumed that this is a good thing to do. The problem is that the intervention of AA/NA is geared to people who are at least in the Contemplation or Preparation stage. Indeed, "the first step of twelve-step programs is to admit that one is powerless over alcohol/drugs/fill in the blank, and that as a result, one's life has become completely unmanageable." This is a profound and humble statement for anyone to make, and it requires a person to be fully aware of their problem. For someone in the Precontemplation stage, there is no likelihood that simply saying those words will be of any clinical utility whatsoever. The person can be directed to the meeting, and they will get some coffee, but it will at best be a pointless exercise. If anything, they will feel out of step with the people in the Action and Maintenance stages around them and end up feeling further alienated.

While the Stages of Change model implied that different treatment approaches needed to be taken for clients at different places along the continuum of change, it remained for another researcher, William R. Miller, the creator of the Motivational Interviewing approach, to elucidate those stage-specific strategies. DiClemente and Miller have stated that the Stages of Change model and Motivational Interviewing grew up simultaneously. This is indeed what happened. DiClemente and Miller met at conferences in the early 1980s and began years of dialogue and informal collaboration. An early result of that collaboration was the 1986 book *Treating Addictive Behaviors: Processes of Change*, which Miller and a colleague edited.

Miller's Motivational Interviewing approach evolved from his work with problem drinkers in the summer of 1973. In his doctoral psychology training, Miller was thrown onto a VA ward in Milwaukee for people suffering from alcoholism. Like me, Miller had no particular training or experiences with people who abuse substances. Unlike me, Miller fell back on something useful, specifically Carl Rogers's client-centered therapy, which involves listening—really listening—to clients and letting them take the lead in the therapeutic process, with only gentle direction from the therapist. Miller has said about Rogers's approach: "Rogers was life-changing for me, both in terms of the counseling style and the way I want to live."[4] The client-centered approach seemed to work. The patients enjoyed being heard, and Miller learned a lot about what bothered them and what held them back.

Without ever really realizing it, Miller developed an empathic listening approach, which centered on ambivalence about change. Miller's ignorance of substance abuse treatment was a blessing. Until very recently, approaches to substance abusers have typically been punitive, coercive, and confrontational, "all for their own good." Miller returned to the University of Oregon and wrote his dissertation on problem drinking. In doing his due diligence on the extant literature, he discovered the people described in the research were not at all like the people he met on the wards: "They were described as lying and incorrigible, defensive and angry," Miller told me. Miller began to write of his different approach, of the empathic approach in therapy in general. His research showed that empathy was a strong predictor of successful outcome.

It wasn't until 1991 that Miller fully articulated his approach, along with a colleague, the Australian Steve Rollnick—although the basic ideas were in place as early as 1983. According to Miller, MI is "a directive, client-centered counseling style for eliciting behavior change by helping clients to explore and resolve ambivalence." As with DiClemente, Miller and colleagues conceived of an entirely new way of looking at ambivalence and motivation. Miller's approach was that ambivalence about substance abuse (and changing any problematic behavior) is a normal state. There are positive reasons to engage in even the most pathological of behaviors. Drugs make one feel very, very good, at least for a short time. And even depression, anxiety, and obsession have their benefits: a feeling that one is uniquely sensitive or special, "a rush" of adrenaline, enjoying the attention on the part of caregivers and family that sometimes attends the process of suffering. "Ambivalence takes the form of a conflict between two courses of action (e.g., indulgence versus restraint), each of which has perceived benefits and costs associated with it." Motivation comes from within the client and is not imposed upon the client by the therapist. The process of Motivational Interviewing involves eliciting the client's own readiness to change. Miller is emphatic that direct persuasion is seldom an effective method for resolving ambivalence. Put more prosaically, when you push people, they tend to push back. Miller says: "It is tempting to try to be helpful by persuading the client of the urgency of the problem and about the benefits of change. However, these tactics generally increase client resistance and diminish the probability of change."

Furthermore, Miller thought of readiness to change not as a client trait but as a fluctuating product of interpersonal interaction. "You can't resist alone on a beach," was how Miller put it to me. Motivation may ultimately reside with the client, but it can also be understood to result from the interactions with the therapist and other people or environmental factors. Motivation to change is typically strongly influenced by family, friends, and community support—or the lack of any of these. As

Miller has summarized, "Internal factors are the basis for change; external factors are the conditions for change."[5] The therapeutic relationship is more like a partnership or companionship than expert-recipient roles.

Before Miller and like-minded colleagues, motivation, particularly in the addictions field, was viewed as a static trait that the client either had or didn't have. As a result, the therapist had little chance of enhancing the client's motivation, and if change did not occur, it was the client's fault. "A client who seemed amenable to clinical advice or accepted the label of alcoholic or drug addict was considered to be motivated, whereas one who resisted a diagnosis or refused to adhere to the proffered treatment was deemed unmotivated."[6] What appeared to be motivation was often superficial compliance. Miller summarized, "Motivation can be understood not as something that one has but rather as something that one does."[7]

Miller developed some formal principles of the MI approach, beyond the general emphasis on expressing empathy and not being confrontational. Some examples are:

> *Support Self-Efficacy.* Ultimately, the client is in charge. MI encourages clients to develop their own solutions to the problems that they themselves have defined. The client is held responsible for choosing and carrying out actions to change in the MI approach, while counselors focus their efforts on helping the clients stay motivated. There is no "right way" to change, and if a given plan for change does not work, clients are limited only by their own creativity as to the number of other plans that might be tried.

> *Develop Discrepancy.* "Motivation for change occurs when people perceive a discrepancy between where they are and where they want to be."[8] MI counselors work to develop this situation through helping clients examine the discrepancies between their current behavior and future goals. When clients perceive that their current behaviors are not leading toward some

important future goal, they become more motivated to make life changes. Of course, MI counselors do not develop discrepancy at the expense of the other MI principles, but gently and gradually help clients to see how some of their current ways of being may lead them away from, rather than toward, their goals.

Over time, Miller and Rollnick have also developed strategies specifically intended for the opening therapeutic sessions when a client is likely to be less ready for change. A critical one is "reflective listening." Reflective listening sounds simple but actually is, according to Miller, quite a challenging skill to master. Reflective listening involves the therapist's restating what the client has said (and not said) in a way that explores whether the therapist has accurately understood the client's meaning. According to Miller, "reflective listening is a way of checking rather than assuming that you know what is meant."[9]

The following would be a brief example of reflective listening:

CLIENT: I wonder if I'm depressed.

THERAPIST: You're noticing something different?

CLIENT: I have a hard time getting out of bed in the morning; there are too many problems out there. Sometimes I just don't want to be alive.

THERAPIST: Life seems overwhelming to you.

CLIENT: But then I do get out of bed, and then I'm usually okay. I go through my day doing everything I need to do. A lot of times everything seems just fine.

THERAPIST: So that's confusing to you. Sometimes you feel pretty good, and then other times you feel like you can't go on another day, and you wonder whether you are becoming depressed.

CLIENT: Yes, that's about right.

The skilled MI counselor knows when to deploy the different techniques and principles. For example, in the opening sessions, one might simply build rapport, elicit the client's own perceptions of the problem, and provide information about the risks of substance abuse or the problems associated with depression. With an ambivalent client, one might indicate that being ambivalent is a normal state, summarize the client's own self-motivational statements, and promote the client's sense of being in charge. With someone in the Preparation stage, one would clarify the client's own strategies for change and negotiate a treatment plan with them. For someone more ready for change, one would support a realistic view of change and reinforce the importance of staying in recovery. And so on.

Motivational Interviewing is beginning to have broad influence throughout health care. The research base for Motivational Interviewing is formidable. There have been 180 outcome studies to date, for people suffering from conditions as diverse as drug and alcohol abuse, smoking, diabetes, gambling, HIV, eating disorders, anxiety, and depression. Most studies have found that people exposed to Motivational Interviewing as a pretreatment, and sometimes as the treatment itself, experience substantial gains.

Motivational Interviewing seems poised for a "tipping point"—a broad takeoff. Without Miller and Rollnick's ever having marketed the technique (they do have a bare-bones Web site, www.motivationalinterviewing.org), the approach is beginning to spread. There are now a thousand trainers around the world.[10] Every correctional officer in Sweden is being trained in Motivational Interviewing.[11] When I spoke to Dr. Marc Gourevitch, newly appointed as director of general internal medicine at the New York University School of Medicine, he told me that one of the principal goals of his tenure was to disseminate

Motivational Interviewing techniques to physicians working in primary care settings, so that they might more effectively address substance abuse and other unhealthy behaviors. Miller told me, "I continue to be astonished at how rapidly MI is diffusing. It certainly surprised me, even when it took off like a rocket in the addiction field, but the spread into other fields has been amazing to me. It's like riding a huge wave with a definite life of its own."[12]

And of course, it makes all the difference when people are genuinely and internally motivated to do something. As *American Psychologist* put it: "Comparisons between people whose motivation is authentic (self-authored or endorsed) and those who are merely externally controlled typically reveal that the former, relative to the latter, have more interest, excitement, and confidence, which in turn is manifest both as enhanced performance, persistence, and creativity, and as heightened vitality, self-esteem, and general well-being. This is so even when the people have the same level of perceived competence for the activity."[13]

Applications of MI as a preparation for the treatment, or pretreatment, for people suffering from depression hold special promise. Ambivalence and resistance to change can be a particular hallmark of depression, as reflected in the following statement by a depressed woman:

"Not changing means that no one will be pressuring me. I can't stand people always telling me I need to do things differently, be more active, stop crying. I feel so rotten; I just want to let myself be. It's all I can do to just manage my kid's activities. I can't do anything else. I don't want to do anything else."[14]

Any technique that can pull a person toward needed treatment is valuable, and MI has been shown in many trials to be capable of that. In a randomized clinical trial, subjects were depressed, economically disadvantaged, pregnant women who were *not* seeking treatment. Some were assigned to a condition where they received either an MI-style "engagement session" followed by eight therapy sessions or a referral for therapy in the community. Almost three-quarters of the women who went through the engagement session completed a course of therapy, whereas only a quarter of the other women did. There have been other similarly promising studies.[15]

To me, both Stages of Change and Motivational Interviewing have the features common to all really good ideas. They are so simple as to be brilliant. They provide an organizing structure that confirms how the world works. Listening to them, as I did when I first was exposed to the Stages of Change model as a struggling case manager, I thought: Oh yes, I knew that all along. I just didn't know that I knew it.

Last, another form of engagement, called peer engagement, has shown great promise, particularly among people with mental illness. Peer engagement involves the hiring of patients, even those who are severely mentally ill, to engage and teach other patients who are not as far along in the treatment cycle—along the Stages of Change, if you will—as they are. It's another of these ideas that makes sense. People who have "been there" know what it's like and are in a unique position to help. "Peer specialists offer hope because they are walking, talking examples of recovery," said Joseph A. Rogers, president and CEO of the Mental Health Association of Southeastern Pennsylvania.[16] Or, as D. Banks McKenzie, founder of a home for alcoholics, wrote in 1875 about the role that the formerly addicted could play in the lives of the presently addicted: "They fully understand each other's language, thoughts, feelings, sorrows, signs, gripes, and passwords, therefore yield to the influence of their reformed brethren much sooner than to the theorists who speak in order that they may receive applause."[17]

While peer engagement does have some historical roots—Harry Stack Sullivan, who helped develop the aforementioned psychiatric assessment tool to screen soldiers for World War II, hired recovering patients as psychiatric aides on his inpatient unit in the 1920s[18]—there has been a remarkable explosion in the last decade in the number of peer-based interventions. George W. Bush's report on mental health care strongly recommended implementation of peer approaches. (Bush has a strangely progressive track record on mental health, both as governor of Texas and as president.) That recommendation has been heeded. Georgia was the first state to make peer specialists part of its formal system of care. Georgia now has almost four hundred peer specialists, all former patients suffering from severe mental illness and now all regular state employees. Five other states now have Medicaid-reimbursable peer services.[19]

Researchers at Yale have studied the role of patients in helping other patients engage in treatment. (Full disclosure: I worked on this study.) They added peer specialists to what are called Assertive Community Treatment (ACT) teams. The idea of ACT teams, developed in the 1960s, was to bring psychiatric treatment and medical services to those who were incapable of coming for treatment in a hospital or office. ACT teams, composed typically of a social worker, a psychiatrist, and sometimes a paraprofessional, drive around in a van to attempt to help people who are often suffering from psychotic disorders, living in parks and under bridges, and refusing services. The Yale researchers did a randomized clinical trial. Half of the ACT teams remained unchanged; half had a peer engagement specialist—a former patient, often formerly homeless themselves—added to the standard team. Clients who were engaged by peers were more receptive to being contacted, had more contacts with the ACT teams, and felt much more liked, understood, and accepted by the teams that had the peer specialists. Feeling better understood and appreciated positively predicted later motivation for formal treatment for psychiatric and drug problems, including attendance at AA and NA meetings. Over time, patients in the peer condition had increasing contacts with treatment teams, and those in the treatment-as-usual model had decreasing contacts.[20]

In other words, peer engagement appears to be the carrot—rather than the stick—that can push previously disenfranchised people to participate in formal health care and substance abuse treatments. Similar results have been found in other studies. The World Health Organization's 2001 report noted that "patients with mental disorders can be very successful in helping themselves, and peer support has been important in a number of conditions for recovery."[21]

The peer movement, with its emphasis on peer providers who are now stable and who are reaching out to others who are less so, has been a central feature of a broader movement, the "recovery movement" in psychiatry. Perhaps two decades old, the recovery movement—invented largely by former patients—is in its relative infancy, but all the momentum has occurred in the last five to ten years. This has led to a paradigm shift in thinking about mental illness and the role of medications in mental illness. It has turned old beliefs and old systems of care in psychiatry upside down.

It can be argued that the recovery movement began when—much to everybody's surprise—researchers found that people with schizophrenia could actually get better. Until then, no one, from Emil Kraepelin on—Kraepelin was the first person to describe schizophrenia, in clinical terms, about one hundred years ago—believed that was possible. Schizophrenia was considered a death sentence, a condition that just got worse and worse, and for which you had better be removed from society and put away someplace dark and quiet. However, starting in the 1970s, the World Health Organization International Pilot Study on long-term outcomes of schizophrenia found, to everybody's shock, that partial to full recovery from the devastations of schizophrenia was just as common, if not more so, than the chronic, progressively downward, and deteriorating course of the illness as described by Kraepelin.

The studies of Courtenay Harding also proved seminal in developing the recovery movement. Harding studied patients leaving Vermont State Hospital, a state psychiatric hospital, between 1955 and 1960. The 269 patients in the study were "the classic back ward cases . . . diagnosed with chronic schizophrenia and deemed unable to survive outside" the hospital. These patients were the happy recipients of one of the first true deinstitutionalization programs, which was highly unusual if not unprecedented for its day. Rather than being told to just leave the hospital, as most deinstitutionalized patients were, the Vermont patients were afforded a ten-year rehabilitation program in the community, which involved the provision of community housing, vocational programs that led to real employment, education, social supports, and individual treatment planning. These services were provided variously by psychiatrists, nurses, vocational counselors, even sociologists. Harding tracked down all but seven of the original 269 patients in the 1980s, an average of thirty years after they were admitted to the hospital. She thought she knew what she was going to find. "My clinical assessors and I were quite skeptical about finding any kind of recovery, because we'd all been trained in the old model. As a former psychiatric nurse on an inpatient unit, it sure didn't look to me that anyone could get better." She was stunned. Following, interviewing, and observing these patients decades after they left the hospital, she found a remarkable two-thirds were doing very well, experiencing few or no symptoms. They were living and working, often with appropriate supports, in the community.

Thinking that the Vermont cohort was some kind of bizarre aberration, Harding sought to find another group of patients to either confirm or disconfirm what she found. After an exhaustive search, she found a similar group of patients in Maine, who had left the Maine state hospitals. She matched each patient in Vermont to a Maine patient on just about every demographic imaginable—diagnosis, age, sex, length of hospitalization, and so on. What Harding found was that the recovery rate for the Maine cohort was still higher than what Kraepelin and those who followed him would have expected—48 percent—but still significantly lower than that of the patients in Vermont. The ex-patients from Vermont had fewer symptoms, more were working, and on a variety of measures, they were experiencing far better adjustment in the community. Upon further analysis, Harding found that the difference between the two programs, Maine and Vermont, was "community integration." In Vermont, patients leaving the hospital were afforded the supports in the community upon which to base their progress and recovery. The Maine program amounted to giving the patients drugs and checking in with them every once in a while. "The Vermont model was self-sufficiency, rehabilitation, and community integration. The Maine model was meds, maintenance, and stabilization," said Harding.[22]

Through such studies, and by *listening to patients*—instead of *listening to Prozac*—three elements of the recovery movement have been identified consistently.

First, social inclusion is critical to getting better. "It's miraculous how people come back," says psychologist Ronald Bassman, who was diagnosed with schizophrenia as a young man, recovered, and is now involved in patient advocacy efforts at the New York State Office of Mental Health.[23] "If you talk to someone who is doing better, he or she will tell you that someone—a friend, a family member, a pastor, a therapist—reached out with warmth and gentleness and kindness." He adds, "This is not what is typically done in the mental health system."[24]

Larry Davidson, a prolific Yale researcher on the recovery from severe mental illness, has examined the totality of the data and found that the medical model of treatment is flawed. "In the medical model, you take a person with a mental illness, you provide treatment in the hopes of reducing symptoms, and then they are supposed to approximate some notion of normality. Our research shows the opposite. You take a person with a mental illness, you then reduce the discrimination and stigma against them, increase their social roles and participation, which provides them a reason to get better in the first place, and then you provide treatment and support. The issue is not so much making them normal but helping them to get their lives back."[25] Davidson's contention is supported by the provocative finding by a number of independent researchers that schizophrenia outcomes are better in developing countries, where social and family supports are generally greater and where people are far less likely to be excluded from their natural communities.[26]

I have witnessed what Davidson is referring to. When you interview patients about how they got better, rarely do they cite a particular doctor or treatment program or medication. What they talk about is a person who was kind when they were really down; they talk about their child that they wanted to support; they talk about God and spirituality; they talk about something that brought them pleasure even when they were cloaked in pain. Many of these reasons to live—the reasons to get better—are highly personal and idiosyncratic. For William Styron, suffering from the black dog of depression and just about to commit suicide, it was a chance encounter with a piece of music by Brahms, the

Alto Rhapsody. If such beautiful things like it exist in the world, he thought, I don't want to leave it. For people in Harding's study, no doubt, it was the desire to live a life outside the hospital.

The second insight gleaned from the recovery movement is that recovery can exist within the context of illness. In other words, recovery does not mean cure. It means living with the illness, managing it, and getting better within certain limitations. "I define recovery as the development of new meaning and purpose as one grows beyond the catastrophe of mental illness," says William Anthony, director of Boston University's Center for Psychiatric Rehabilitation. "My feeling is you can have episodic symptoms and still believe and feel you're recovering. It is a matter of moving beyond the debilitating phases of the illness."[27]

That recovery does not usually mean the removal of all symptoms represents a novel and distinctly un-American way of looking at psychiatric illness, and at illness in general. We like to think of the destination rather than the journey; this is the journey as the destination. Generally, medicine defines recovery, or likes to define recovery, as the removing of all symptoms, as if they were toxic and foreign entities having nothing to do with us. In fact, many common illnesses—diabetes, HIV/AIDS, forms of hepatitis, cardiovascular disease—do not conform to that model whatsoever. The fact remains that most major psychiatric illnesses are episodic but chronic. The medications, as we have learned, are a long way from providing any true remediation of even major psychiatric disorders. Recovery then involves both a coming to terms with symptoms—one hopes in the context of their gradual moderation, but this is not always the case—and finding a meaningful life in their midst. For many patients, this is a decades-long process of acceptance and resolve. At the end of the process, some patients can actually say they are glad they have experienced an illness, within reason, as it has enriched their lives and appreciation of things beyond measure. (One has to be careful with such sentiments not to romanticize the suffering of illness. Nonetheless, it is a common statement made by those who find meaning in the face of ongoing symptoms.) As a reflection of this embrace, or at least acceptance, of symptoms, one finds in the recovery movement a refreshing and sometimes disarming honesty about the problems people have to face day in and day out. Web sites created by members of the recovery movement are called such things as www.psychosissucks.com and are organized by entities like "The Madness Group." There is also the recovery movement–friendly "Bonkers Institute for Nearly Genuine Research, whose motto is "Advancing in the general direction of bona fide science since last Tuesday" at www.bonkersinstitute.org.

A further lesson learned is that getting better requires identifying the patient's strengths and resources as well as his weaknesses (usually known as symptoms or diagnosis). This is again a departure from the standard medical model, which is based on "chief complaint," "presenting problems, and "symptoms" as the sole framework or guide for the treatment. Medicine is simply not used to thinking about assets and resources. It is a problem-solving discipline, and therefore, it has mainly been involved with everything that's wrong with a person. Psychiatrist George Vaillant, of Harvard, reviewed abstracts of all the scholarly psychological and psychiatric articles published between 1987 and 2002 and found 57,800 articles on anxiety and 70,856 on depression. But only 5,701 mentioned "life satisfaction," and only 851 mentioned "joy."[28]

In reaction to this, so-called recovery-oriented treatment plans in progressive psychiatric programs place the patients' resources and abilities—their resilience—on par with, or with even greater emphasis than, their problems. The idea is to look at what's right with a person in addition to, or even more than, what's wrong with them. This makes a great deal of sense. In my work with patients suffering from mental illness, I have found the critical pathway to health is not typically the robustness of the disease, but the resources of the person to deal with the affliction. Erik Erikson put it a slightly different way: "We cannot even really know what causes neurotic suffering until we have an idea of what causes real health. This we have only begun to investigate."[29]

Social service agencies, which exist on the margins of psychiatry and medicine but often treat the sickest patients with the least amount of resources, are always in dire need of tools that work. Partly out of desperation, social service agencies are often the earliest adopters of progressive developments in the field, like Motivational Interviewing, well before they hit the medical establishment. But it's not only desperation. Social service agencies are increasingly under pressure from government funders and public managed-care entities to quantitatively demonstrate the statistical value of their services. As a result, when social service agencies find something that works, they use it. At good agencies it is now standard practice to make services and treatment plans "strength-based." So if the goal is to get a job for a client living in a halfway house, the plan would be to first identify all the strengths and abilities that the client has in order to achieve the goal. The other approach is to have the client put the goal in his own words. What you find is that when clients themselves identify what they want to do and the strengths they have to actually do it, the outcomes are dramatically better.

The final aspect of the recovery movement, and in this it has a great deal in common with the Stages of Change model and Motivational Interviewing, is that the *patient is in charge and is the ultimate expert in his own recovery*. As Larry Davidson (and Home Depot) puts it: "You can do it; we can help." Along with Courtenay Harding, John Strauss, professor emeritus of psychiatry and my mentor at Yale, was one of the early researchers to show that people with schizophrenia could actually get better.

A turning point occurred about 1985. Strauss was interviewing a patient, based on a structured interview, when the woman stopped him and said: "Why don't you ever ask me what I do to help myself?"[30]

This led to a paradigm shift in John's thinking. From that time, his research has become much more qualitative (less statistical and more exploratory) and evolved in mutual collaboration with his research subjects, or participants. They can teach him about their worlds and what they do to make sense of them. John has spent much of his retirement writing about patients as people rather than carriers of symptoms, and teaching colleagues to do the same. John's transformation has not always been well received by colleagues. After he gave one of his newer papers at a scientific meeting in New York, a psychiatrist said: "But, John, you used to do such good work!"

This negative reception is not surprising. Listening to patients cuts against the establishment grain. We live in an age of experts, where we cede control of our bodies and our being to others. Different parts of our bodies go to different experts. It is sacrilegious, medically speaking, to think that one could be the expert on one's self—while also valuing and seeking the expertise of professionals.

Since Harding, researchers based primarily at Dartmouth have developed a series of empirically validated "illness management" techniques, in which people with even the most severe mental illnesses like schizophrenia take charge of their own recovery, by setting goals, completing workbooks, making critical treatment decisions (such as health care proxy decisions should they become psychotic), and so on. Some of these illness management tool kits pertain to medications, but most don't, addressing instead, social support, vocational skills, recreation, and life "outside the illness."[31] These tool kits have been endorsed and are distributed by SAMHSA the federal government's substance abuse and mental health services administration.

Mary Ellen Copeland was diagnosed with bipolar disorder at age thirty-seven. She was given pills—pills that she was told she would need to take for the rest of her life—until she developed a toxic reaction to them. She has written:

> During the time I was taking the medication I could have been learning to manage my moods. I could have been learning that relaxation and stress reduction techniques and fun activities can help reduce the symptoms . . . In the years since then, I have reached out to many other sources for help and guidance. They include:
>
> - a nutritionist who told me that I needed more B vitamins and some amino acids,

- a minister who felt my problems would be eased by more involvement in a religious community—that I was out of touch with God,
- various counselors who told me I should try to heal my relationship with my husband, or that I should leave my husband, and tried to direct me in and out of other relationships,
- a body worker who told me that my healing was dependent on the thoroughness with which I could remember and share childhood trauma,
- a family member who told me that I should "pull myself up by the bootstraps,"
- a well-meaning friend who said I should go home and bake pies for my family,
- a benefits provider that accused me of malingering and being noncompliant.

When I told a psychiatrist that I wanted to write a book, he told me that I was being "grandiose." Since then I have written 10 books and had them published. The same psychiatrist told me I could never lead a workshop. Since then I have led hundreds of workshops—attended by thousands of people—all over the world.

The most important lesson that I learned from all of this is that in making decisions about me and my life, I first must listen to myself. I must ask myself what I know and feel about myself. Then, if I want to, I can reach out to others for their ideas. As each of them shares their opinion or gives their advice, I can weigh it carefully and see how it resonates with me—does it feel right to me or doesn't it? If it feels right I can do or believe as they suggest. If it doesn't feel right, I don't need to.[32]

Mary Ellen Copeland became the author of *The Wellness Recovery Action Plan* (WRAP), a client-centered, strength-based workbook that patients suffering from mental illness complete in order to be the author of their own recovery. WRAP has been wildly successful and is used nationally, including at VA hospitals.

Fortunately, today in psychiatry there is an array of treatment choices available: psychoanalysis, CBT, medication, diet, exercise, self-management, peer support. Increasingly, it should be the initial and primary job of psychiatry to educate the patient about all the treatment options available. The patient, as expert in the self, will make the choice, in conjunction with the psychiatrist, psychologist, or social worker, who will act as an expert consultant. This, I suggest, is the new model for mental health treatment.

The totality of these alternative and human approaches is catching on. In late 2004, the National Institute for Health and Clinical Excellence (NICE) in Britain, which is charged with advising the National Health Service on best practices, issued a formal guide of Clinical Guidelines for Depression.[33] The following were their recommendations, in order, for the treatment of mild and moderate depression:

1. *Sleep and Anxiety Management*
2. *Watchful Waiting.* A recommendation of further assessment in two weeks, recognizing that some mild depressions clear up without intervention.
3. *Exercise.* "Patients of all ages with mild depression should be advised of the benefits of following a structured and supervised program of typically up to three sessions a week, for between ten to twelve weeks."
4. *Guided Self-Help.* "A self-administered intervention . . . which makes use of a range of books or a self-help manual," often based on CBT principles.
5. *CBT, Brief Counseling, Problem-Solving Therapy.* "In both mild to moderate depression, psychological treatment specifically focused on depression (such as problem-solving therapy, brief CBT and counseling) of six to eight sessions over ten to twelve weeks should be considered."

The recommendations conclude with a discussion of antidepressant drugs:

> 6. The recommendation for antidepressants is only when the depression persists after psychological and lifestyle interventions have been tried. "Antidepressants are not recommended for the initial treatment of mild depression, because the risk-benefit ratio is poor."

With that last sentence, the era of cosmetic and frivolous psychopharmacology has started to come to an end, and the Serotonin Empire underwent an attack that shook it at its very foundation.

It remains for Americans, and for the American psychiatric establishment, to be as forward-thinking as their British counterparts. Such a reverse exchange would seem somehow to be appropriate: American companies get wealthy importing the drugs to Britain, and in return, the British offer wise counsel on how we can manage our anxiety and depression.

CHAPTER SEVEN

The Sea Snail Syndrome

Finally, the other reason we should pay attention to psychosocial approaches is that it is no longer tenable to dismiss them as soft and mushy-headed. In perhaps the most ironic development of the neuro-revolution, psychotherapy and, indeed, social experience have been shown to change the brain at a structural and functional level in a way that can be comparable to drugs.

A sea snail, albeit a giant marine one, *Aplysia californica*, proved it. The lessons gleaned from *Aplysia* have ignited a revolution in psychiatry and are already leading to a merger between biological and social psychiatry, between medication and psychotherapy, mind and brain.

Aplysia has a long and distinguished history with natural historians. The animal was first mentioned by Pliny the Elder, the Roman natural philosopher and author of *Naturalis Historia*. In *The Voyage of the Beagle*, Charles Darwin wrote of *Aplysia:* "This sea-slug is about five inches long; and is of a dirty-yellowish color, veined with purple . . . It feeds on the delicate seaweeds . . . This slug, when disturbed, emits a very fine purplish-red fluid, which stains the water for the space of a foot around."

Aplysia have a soft body and no outer shell and are sometimes called sea hares because of their resemblance to rabbits; *Aplysia californica*, so named because they are found off the coast of California, grow to about a foot long. In the wild, the saving grace of *Aplysia* is that it tastes very bad. It has been said that its principal predator is the neurobiologist.[1]

There's a simple reason why *Aplysia* is so beloved by scientists. It has a small number of cells, and the cells that it does have are magnificently large. Its brain has about 20,000 cells, compared to the approximately 100 billion in the mammalian brain. Some of *Aplysia*'s cells are one millimeter in diameter, making them visible to the naked eye and allowing for the relatively easy insertion of microelectrodes to record electrical activity.[2]

Aplysia's keeper in the lab for the last four decades has been the psychiatrist Eric Kandel. Kandel's relationship with the humble sea snail can only be described as an ongoing love affair—and a particularly rewarding one, resulting in Kandel's winning the Nobel Prize in Physiology or Medicine in 2000. Kandel has said: "I periodically think about abandoning *Aplysia*, and every time my wife will say that I'm crazy—that I can't give it up. She is right. I continue to find such interesting things in that animal! . . . there is no other model system in all of biology that comes close to *Aplysia* for studying the movement of substances from the cell body to the synapse and the flux of signals from the synapse to the cell body."[3]

Kandel's personal history embodies what he argues for in his work, the intertwining and ultimate blending of science and human experience. Born in Vienna, where his father owned a small toy store, he grew up in a neighborhood not far from Freud's apartment. His childhood was relatively undisturbed until there was the proverbial knock on the door. Men who identified themselves as Nazi police whisked the family out and forced them to stay with strangers. The family ultimately got out of Austria, arriving in Brooklyn in 1939.

In the United States, Kandel was able to access social and educational circles that would likely not have been available to him had he stayed in Austria. As an undergraduate at Harvard, he met the children of other Viennese, some of whose parents had been psychoanalysts. "Through them I got extremely interested in psychoanalysis, and changed my career interests from history and literature," which he had studied as an undergraduate at Harvard. In medical school, Kandel's growing interest in biological psychiatry shifted him to neuroscience, then in its infancy. "I thought I should learn something about the brain, because an analyst should know something about what's between the ears."[4] By the mid-1950s, he had set his sights on uncovering a biological basis for Freud's concepts of ego, id, and superego. Kandel would be the first to admit that his grandiose ambition was reflected by another psychological construct—hubris. If that was what he wanted to do, he was advised by his Columbia mentor, Harry Grundfest, to do it "one cell at a time."[5]

Kandel believed that since nothing was known about the basic cell biology of learning and behavior, the place to start was with animals, and the simpler the better. He intuited that the basic structure of learning and behavior was shared across species, and the analysis of learning at the cellular level would reveal a "universal mechanism." But in the 1950s and 1960s, it was widely believed that simple animal models were of little to no relevance to human brains and behavior. Kandel was warned that veering off on such a tangent would significantly damage his career.[6]

Having found *Aplysia*, the undeterred Kandel had a seemingly simple question: "What happens in the brain of an animal when it actually learns a task? How does it remember?"[7] Somehow Kandel sensed, as he put it in an interview, "that a cellular approach would open up new techniques to address complicated problems, and I think my good fortune was to apply this to learning and memory at a time when no one was thinking in those terms."[8]

Kandel applied Pavlovian and Skinnerian principles to his study of *Aplysia*, specifically the concepts of habituation and sensitization. Habituation is the process by which an animal gradually learns to disregard a stimulus; in sensitization, on the other hand, the animal responds in a heightened way to a previously neutral stimulus after something noxious occurs. To study these, Kandel focused on a simple behavior in *Aplysia*, the gill-withdrawal response. If one prods *Aplysia* anywhere near its gill, the animal withdraws and folds a flap of skin over it for protection. The more you do it, the less vigorously the sea snail responds. The snail gets used to the prodding—it habituates. To model sensitization, Kandel applied a strong shock to either the head or the tail. The snails responded to the intensity of the stimulus, and in its aftermath, produced a more rapid and exaggerated gill-withdrawal reflex in response to the same light touch near the gill. The snails soon learned to avoid the shocks or became hypersensitive to them, developing, arguably, the snail equivalent of anxiety. This meant they had developed primitive memories for the shocks.

To Kandel's surprise, he was able to track the changes in the synaptic connections between the cells affected by these stimuli. By inserting a microelectrode into a cell and then sending an electrical signal into nearby cells, he was able to identify the affected *presynaptic cells*, the neurons that were sending electrical and chemical signals to other neurons across the synapse. In Kandel's words, "Thus it proved possible for the first time in any animal to map the working synaptic connections between individual cells, which I could use as a method for working out the neural circuit controlling a behavior."[9] In other words, he found the neurons and motor cells that produced the movement in the gill.

Kandel saw that synapses between neurons could easily and systematically be altered in response to stimulation. The changes were remarkable. "New growth of synapses occurs in front of your eyes over the course of a day," Kandel has said.[10] "In *Aplysia*," he says, "you can see in front of your eyes that the connections change. When the animal remembers something for the long term, it grows new synaptic connections."[11] He learned further that habituation weakened the synapse, and sensitization strengthened it by the creation of new proteins.

Kandel writes, "This suggested that synaptic plasticity is built into the very nature of the chemical synapse, its molecular architecture. In the broadest terms it suggested that the flow of information in the various neural circuits of the brain could be modified by learning."[12] Learning is nothing more than the strengthening of connections between neurons. In other words, the brain of *Aplysia* was physically changed by experience. More specifically, experience can determine which of many genes are expressed. As Columbia University neuroscientist Norman Doidge wrote, "Kandel's work demonstrates that the common metaphor that compares the mind to a computer, with unmodifiable hardware (a brain) and malleable software (thoughts, memories), is wrong. Rather, thought can actually change the structure of the brain; the software modifies the hardware.[13] Kandel hadn't found where the id, ego, and superego were located, but he did discover the universal principle that he was after. He demonstrated the molecular basis of learning, and even more broadly, he had demonstrated the *plasticity* of the nervous system.

So plastic are our brains that research over the last decade has shown that at least some part of the brain is capable of growing new neurons, which for a century had been thought to be impossible. Scientists had believed that the regenerative capacities of our bodies did not extend to the central nervous system—the brain and the spinal cord. The immutability of the brain was one of the central dogmas of neuroscience.

Kandel is among many investigators of neuroplasticity, but he is about the only one who has fully articulated its implications for creating an extraordinarily simple but all-inclusive vision of psychiatry. He has written eloquently that the concept that we are controlled by genes—or, as I think it can be conceived in the popular mindset, our neurons, neurochemistry, a "chemical imbalance"—is "fundamentally wrong."[14] In a seminal article, 1998's "A New Intellectual Framework for Psychiatry," Kandel explains that, contrary to popular understanding, genes are not the unchanging controllers of behavior. Kandel reminds us that there are two functions of genes, only one of which is beyond social or individual control. Genes have a template function, which is simply the ability to provide succeeding generations with copies of themselves. The fidelity in this replication process is very high; it cannot be altered by social processes of any sort; and it can be changed only by mutation, which is rare and usually random. In the popular imagination, as we have seen, the role of genes begins and ends there, and we are impotent in the face of the inevitable, predetermined, and unmodifiable actions of the genes.

But, as Kandel points out, genes have another function, a transcriptional function, which is the ability of a gene to direct the manufacture of specific proteins in any given cells, the expression of which makes a brain cell a brain cell and a liver cell a liver cell. Although almost every cell of the body has all of the genes that are present in every other cell, in any given cell type only a fraction of genes, perhaps 10 percent to 20 percent, are expressed through the transcriptional function. The other genes are effectively silent. A liver cell is a liver cell and a brain cell is a brain cell only because these cell types express different subsets of the total population of genes they possess.

The transcriptional function of genes is responsive to environmental factors. Specifically, internal and external stimuli—such as steps in the development of the brain, hormones, stress, learning and social interaction, the prodding of the gill of *Aplysia*—change how genes are expressed. Kandel writes: "The regulation of gene expression by social factors makes all bodily functions, including all functions of the brain, susceptible to social influences." The difficulty is that people, even scientists, confuse these two functions of genes. Kandel has said, "People who are not scientists think that genes are the ultimate controllers of behavior, but what they don't realize is that environment can alter the expression of genes and thereby modify the anatomical structure of the brain—and of course, *Aplysia* was the first to reveal that."[15] To think that the sole function of genes is the template function—the inexorable transmission of hereditary information from one generation to another—is "fatalistic" and "fundamentally wrong," as well as dangerous, leading to the eugenics movements of the 1920s and 1930s.

It is astonishing to consider that what we think and what we do influences genetic transcription.[16] It takes us out of the realm of genetic determinism that has so dominated the mind-set of recent years. But in the wondrous glow of the latest fMRI and the latest report on the genetic basis of some new disorder, this complex, nuanced, and ultimately hopeful message has tragically not yet entered public awareness, even though it affects our daily lives.

In 2000, researchers at University College in London scanned the brains of London taxi drivers and found that their hippocampi—the hippocampus is the part of the brain associated with memory and navigation—were larger than those of most people. The longer one had been a cabdriver, the larger the hippocampus. London is, of course, a huge city, and becoming a cabdriver requires passing a rigorous examination on its geography and streets after a training period commonly called "doing the knowledge." Clearly, as the lead researcher Dr. Eleanor Maguire said, the hippocampi of the taxi drivers "changed its structure to accommodate their huge amount of navigation experience." (Which led one cabbie to say, "I never noticed part of my brain growing—it makes you wonder what happened to the rest of it.")[17] This is the ultimate pragmatic example of experience-dependent plasticity. Working a part of the brain like a muscle, based on environmental needs, makes it change in structure and function, even size. (On the inverse side, veterans of the Vietnam and Gulf wars who have suffered from trauma have reduced hippocampi. It has been proven that the release of the hormone cortisol, under stress, literally kills cells in the hippocampus.)

All of this goes to show that Shakespeare wasn't so far off the mark when he wrote in *Hamlet:* "There is nothing either good or bad, but thinking makes it so."

It has long been known that when rats are raised in enriched environments (better nutrition, proper nurturing, good diet and rest, environmental stimuli like toys and exercise wheels), they perform much better than controls on learning tasks. Neuroplasticity researchers since Kandel have since found an entire arsenal of neural correlates for that enhanced behavior. Specifically, environmental enrichment and stimulation have been found to augment all of the following: the weight of the brain, the thickness of the cortex, the number and activity of glial cells, the size of the cell body and nucleus of neurons, the branching (the growth) of dendrites, the density of the spines of dendrites, and the number of new neurons in the hippocampus.[18]

Furthermore, it has been shown that these various brain changes transpire only in the part of the brain in which the task is learned. This illustrates that the proper types of stimulation during development and beyond lead to long-lasting brain changes and enhancements in learning. As if we needed further proof, these studies provide a biological explanation for the efficacy of early childhood social and educational programs.[19]

The most immediately applicable implication of Kandel's work is also exquisitely ironic. Neuroplasticity supports the efficacy of old-fashioned psychotherapy, which, of course, has continued to decline in the age of the Serotonin Empire. Who would have thought neuroscience would show that psychotherapy is a robust treatment capable of working at a biological level?

As proof, Kandel (and others) point to a now famous study of obsessive-compulsive patients. Obsessive-compulsive disorder is associated with functional hyperactivity of the head of the right caudate nucleus (*nucleus* as used here means a larger cluster of neurons, not part of an individual cell). It has been hypothesized that the caudate acts as a sort of filter, blocking extraneous thoughts and impulses, and that in patients with OCD, the filter malfunctions, allowing unwanted thoughts to spill over into consciousness. After effective treatment with either an SSRI *or* with cognitive-behavioral techniques, investigators have found that there is a substantial decrease in this excessive activity in the right caudate nucleus. The stunning result: both psychotherapy and medication change the brain. This finding has been replicated in trials with people suffering from other psychiatric conditions. Paxil and cognitive-behavioral therapy, administered to separate groups of patients, each led to similar changes in the brains of people suffering from depression.[20] Subsequent research has revealed subtle differences in how CBT and antidepressants alter the activity of the brain.[21]

Kandel's writing in "A New Intellectual Framework for Psychiatry" builds to these remarkable statements:

> These arguments suggest that when a therapist speaks to a patient and the patient listens, the therapist is not only making

> eye contact and voice contact, but the action of neuronal machinery in the therapist's brain is having an indirect and, one hopes, long-lasting effect on the neuronal machinery in the patient's brain: and quite likely, vice versa . . . We face the interesting possibility that as brain imaging techniques improve, these techniques might be useful not only for diagnosing various neurotic illnesses but also for monitoring the progress of psychotherapy.[22]

Again, researchers since Kandel have identified highly specific biological changes in the brain unleashed by the process of psychotherapy.

Psychotherapy affects cerebral metabolic rates in the brain. The OCD study described above also showed that psychotherapy and Prozac produced decreased cerebral metabolic rates in the right caudate nucleus. Additionally, imaging studies of patients diagnosed with posttraumatic stress disorder found that psychotherapy increased prefrontal metabolism and decreased limbic system activation in the brain.

In broad terms, this means that psychotherapy enhanced activity in the part of the brain associated with executive function—judgment, decision-making, rationality—and subdued activity in the part of the brain that processes emotion, fear, and aggressive instincts. For people suffering from PTSD, this would appear to be a good thing.

Psychotherapy affects serotonin metabolism in the brain. Finnish researchers have showed that psychotherapy may have a significant impact on serotonin metabolism. Researchers imaged the brain of a twenty-five-year-old man suffering from borderline personality disorder and depression before he started a year of psychotherapy. Another man with the same diagnoses also underwent brain imaging but received no psychotherapy or treatment of any kind. The initial imaging of the men showed that they both had significantly reduced serotonin uptake in parts of their brain when compared with ten healthy control subjects. Imaging one year later showed that the man who had received one year of therapy had developed normal serotonin uptake, while the control patient continued to have significantly impaired serotonin uptake. As the patient who received psychotherapy took no medication as part of his treatment, the finding suggests that it was the therapy itself that may have normalized his serotonin metabolism.[23]

The limits of neuroplasticity are unclear, but there is no longer any doubt that psychotherapy results in detectable changes in the brain.[24] Psychotherapy can be conceived as a process of manipulating and exploiting brain plasticity. Not only that, some researchers of schizophrenia have been reconceiving mental illness as a disease that results from dysfunction in synaptic plasticity. Its remediation would then involve enhancing plasticity. Indeed, Steven Arnold, a psychiatrist at the University of Pennsylvania's Laboratory for Cellular and Molecular Neuropathology, has said: "If anybody would pay for it, techniques to enhance plasticity would be the ideal treatment for schizophrenia. They would include speech therapy, cognitive therapy, and exercises, the teaching of life skills, and techniques to address distortions in thinking.[25]

Indeed, intriguing work at the University of Minnesota has shown just this. "There is neuroplasticity even in the prefrontal cortex. The prefrontal cortex is the corner office of the brain, where all those important executive decisions are made about what to attend to and how to reach goals," according to Angus MacDonald III, a clinical psychologist and cognitivie neuroscientist at the University of Minnesota. "People with schizophrenia, who generally have difficulty implementing these functions, can, with practice, improve their functioning in these brain regions." While these changes are subtle, they are substantial enough to be observable by using functional MRI.

Call it the "Sea Snail syndrome." Psychiatry has long been a house divided against itself,[26] plagued by a series of false dichotomies: Mind versus Brain, Genes versus Environment, Medication versus Psychotherapy, the artsy soft-nosed therapists versus the macho hard-nosed scientists, Psychology versus Psychiatry, Social versus Biological, Left Brain versus Right Brain, and on and on.

There has been a destructive, simplistic oscillation between these polarities, a well-established dichotomy. It goes back at least to Sir Francis Galton, who wrote in *English Men of Science: Their Nature and Nurture*, in 1874:

> The phrase "nature and nurture" is a convenient jingle of words, for it separates under two distinct heads the innumerable elements of which personality is composed . . . When nature and nurture compete for supremacy on equal terms . . . the former proves to be the stronger.[27]

The pendulum then swung so far back the other way, during the psychoanalytic era, to a total disregard for genetics. In 1948, a visiting Danish psychiatrist found that most of his American colleagues would not even discuss the possibility of genetic causes of mental disorders. Psychoanalysis had become the scientific religion of choice.[28] (And beyond that, genetics, in the aftermath of Nazi experiments, had become a bad religion.) And now we are way back to Galton. When in doubt, genes are the cause.

But *Aplysia* has told us that in one stroke, we can do away of all these artificial distinctions. "Nature and nurture stand in reciprocity, not opposition," as Harvard psychiatrist Leon Eisenberg has written.[29] The Sea Snail syndrome is the opportunity for psychology and neuroscience to mutually inform each other, in Kandel's phrase, "*interactively and synergistically, not only additively.*"

Indeed, the nuanced and sophisticated field of social neuroscience has begun just recently to emerge.[30] The first references, in the early 1990s, that such a field could actually exist were greeted with disdain. "There was a lot of skepticism among neuroscientists about studying anything outside the cranium," says John Cacioppo, director of the Center for Cognitive and Social Neuroscience at the University of Chicago. The link between brains and social behavior was just too far to go. But with today's tools it's starting to be possible. "Today we can start to make sense of how the brain drives social behavior and in turn how our social world influences our brain and biology," says Cacioppo.[31]

Social neuroscience is one of the most dynamic areas in science. The field's first conference was held at UCLA in 2001. Seventy people were expected to attend, but three hundred showed up. Since the early 2000s, the National Institutes of Health has dedicated millions to fund pilot research.[32] There are new graduate programs opening and money flowing from major foundations (the John D. and Catherine T. MacArthur Foundation's Network on Mind-Body Interactions, the James S. McDonnell Foundation's "Bridging Mind, Brain and Behavior)." The field's own journal, *Social Neuroscience*, was launched in 2006.

Although the field has only recently begun to gain some traction, some prescient researchers have been working in this area since the 1970s. At that time, researchers at the University of Southern California undertook an intriguing and ambitious study of children in Mauritius, an independent island nation off the east coast of Africa in the Indian Ocean. The idea of this study was to see if there was a way to prevent two major mental disorders: schizophrenia and antisocial disorder. Antisocial disorder leads to a great deal of criminal behavior and is marked by aggression, impulsivity, and lack of remorse. The study began in 1972 and 1973 when the children were three years old. Children from two towns in Mauritius were assigned to two groups. One hundred children were placed in an experimental "enrichment program"; a control group of about 350 children received no additional services. The enrichment group and the control group were matched on ten variables, including ethnicity, gender, age, nutritional status, cognitive ability, temperament, parental social class, mother's age at birth. The children began the enrichment program at three years of age and participated just two years, until age five. The enrichment program took place at two new, well-appointed elementary schools that were built specifically for the study, and where the student-teacher ratio was about one teacher for five students. There were three key elements to the intervention: nutrition, education, and exercise. Children in the enrichment program drank milk and ate mutton, fish, or chicken and salad daily. The educational program focused on verbal skills, visual-spatial skills, memory, and the development of conceptual thinking. A variety of learning modes were offered to the children, and they included the use of toys, art, handicrafts, and music. Children in the enrichment program were engaged in physical activity an average of two and a half hours a day, a regimen that included gymnastics, outdoor sports, and free play. There were field trips, walks, instruction in basic hygiene, and medical check-ins every two months. Staff at the nursery schools was trained in nutrition, hygiene, anatomy, and childhood disorders and illnesses. The children in the control condition, on the other hand, went through the typical Mauritian school experience, with the usual grade-school curriculum and a teacher-student ratio of one to thirty. No exercise program was provided. For lunch children generally ate the standard diet: bread only, rice and bread, or rice only.

The researchers returned to Mauritius in 1987, when the research subjects were seventeen years old. The researchers did inventories that probed for antisocial personality disorder and personality disorder and assembled a comprehensive data set on behavior problems. (Schizotypal personality disorder is considered a precursor for the later development of schizophrenia and is marked by flatness in mood, suspiciousness, reduced capacity, and various cognitive distortions if not delusions.) The researchers found that at age seventeen, those in the enriched groups had significantly lower scores on indicators of schizotypal personality and lower scores on cognitive disorganization. Students in the control group had much higher levels of excessive motor activity, psychotic behavior, and conduct disorder. Six years later, the court records reflecting involvement with the legal system were dramatically different between the two groups. At age twenty-three, 3 of 83 children in the enriched protocol had a legal record, as opposed to 35 of the 355 in the control condition.

In reviewing the outcomes, the researchers couldn't identify which of the elements of the enriched program may have been the critical factor: nutrition, education, or exercise. However, the three-year-olds who started off malnourished had significantly better later outcomes (at age seventeen and twenty-three) as a result of the enrichment program than those who were not malnourished when they were three years old. The researchers wondered if the omega-3 fatty acids in the fish might be significant as a moderator and improver of behavior. The researchers speculated that the exercise programs may have benefited the children's brain structure.[33] This has been established by experiments with mice. Mice that run in cages experience a growth of brain cells, and mice that run in cages together with other mice experience even greater growth of brain cells.[34] It is reasonable to assume that the more intensive and enriched educational experience enhanced the intricacy and increased the number of synaptic connections in the brains of the children. If mental illnesses are diseases partially of synaptic plasticity, the enhanced learning may have been a protective factor as well.

Diet, exercise, and learning acted as prophylactics against the development of mental illness. More than previously thought, some of the answers lie in the simple, low-tech techniques readily available to us.

And the following story shows how a full embrace of psychosocial and neuroscientific knowledge, working in concert, can do no less than save one person's life:

Depending on the day, if not the hour, Rex believed he was either an assistant district attorney or Moses. The legal part of the delusion was highly specific—it wasn't a district attorney but an *assistant* district attorney that Rex believed himself to be. Rex also very much liked to smoke crack and spent most of his days either smoking it or engaged in the activities necessary to acquire it. He favored neon-colored polyester suits as well and kept one side of his head perfectly shaved, while the other side grew into long reddish blond locks. He often sprinted down Chapel Street in New Haven barefoot with a boom box in the January snow, in search of the Holy Ghost, the perfect vial, or whatever else inhabited his psychotic universe.

Rex lived at "the Barracks," so called because it was once an armory. In its current incarnation, the Barracks, located on the wrong side of the tracks in New Haven, is a "mental health" shelter. It is the temporary home to thirty psychotic and homeless men. (Or not so temporary: lengths of stay among its residents range from a few days to seven years.) The Barracks looks like a rundown, sprawling Gothic castle, complete with turrets. One wouldn't be surprised to see a moat around it. As it is, there is a security station, with metal detectors, where the men are searched and scanned as they go in and out all day long.

At the Barracks, Rex slept in a metal bunk bed in one of a dozen dark gray dorm rooms, all along the linoleum-tiled hallways. Men paced up and down these hallways, muttering imprecations to themselves. One man spent most of the time inside the bathroom and had done so for five years. Another spent his days sitting in a chair, covering his ears and trying to block out the voices. Inside the shelter there was also a medical clinic, a dental clinic, a psychiatric clinic (with doctors, substance abuse counselors, and case managers), a hair salon, a TV and game room, an extremely popular smoking room, and a once distinguished, now dilapidated oak-paneled dining room with an oddly collegiate atmosphere. However, what detracted from the atmosphere of conviviality and fellowship was the fact that the men hardly spoke to one another at meals. The residents of the Barracks were far more likely to talk to themselves or sit in a sort of dull unmoving oblivion as they ate.

At least initially, Rex had no interest in the amenities of the shelter. He cut his own hair—or at least half of his hair—and therefore didn't need the salon. He refused all medications and eluded the psychiatric staff whenever possible. Rex preferred to spend the day running, often literally, through the streets of New Haven, in search of jobs—he was always looking for work but never got any—and crack and God. His only contact with the shelter staff was his perfunctory daily attendance at the morning meeting, which he attended only because the staff gave out a free cigarette afterwards.

One day, however, after Rex had lived at the Barracks for about six months, something in a psychiatric clinic's office caught his eye. It was a yellow legal pad upon which a staff member was writing notes. Rex asked the staff member, José, if he could have a legal pad and was told that he could. From that time on, Rex loved yellow legal pads, because on the days, and hours, that he believed himself to be an assistant district attorney, the fact that he had a legal pad proved that he was one. Rex carried legal pads with him everywhere and scribbled down copious notes about his activities and thoughts as he roamed the streets. He came into the clinic daily, picked up a legal pad, and left as quickly as he could.

After Rex had been collecting legal pads daily for a couple of months, José took him aside and said gently, in heavily accented English: "Look, Rex, the program doesn't have much money. We can't afford to give you all these legal pads. We can give you one more legal pad, but we'd really appreciate it if you keep it here in the program." José, who understands trouble—a medical doctor by training, he came to the Barracks from Guatemala, where he was almost assassinated for his leftist political activities—had a plan. The legal pad ploy was his way of enticing Rex into treatment at the clinic. Rex, who was always affable even when floridly psychotic, said sure, and from that time on, he came daily to the clinic to be—simply to be—in the presence of his beloved legal pad. At first Rex just sat in the dayroom clutching his pad and stared off into space, or slept, or paced, but after a while that got boring and he inevitably started to take notice of the numerous activities at the clinic such as the daily groups held on medications, substance abuse, education about mental illness, parenting, and so on. For the first time, Rex ventured into the room where all these meetings were held, and over time he became one of the most consistent attendees, all the while holding his pad. Over time he responded in particular to the group on substance abuse. By simple virtue of the fact that he was spending less time on the street and more time hearing about the liabilities of crack, Rex began cutting back on his usage. In a surprisingly short time he stopped using crack altogether. And when he stopped taking crack, he started taking medications. The clinic psychiatrist put him on the antipsychotic medication Haldol.

Haldol worked like a charm. Rex is one of the lucky ones—those 20 percent of people with schizophrenia for whom the drugs seem to stop the most visible symptoms in their tracks. The "half-life" of Haldol is about a week. ("Half-life" is the time it takes for half the medication to leave the body, an indicator of how long it takes for the agent to have a therapeutic effect.) Sure enough, after about a week, Rex seemed to settle down. The suits got less wild; the delusions seemed to dissipate; he shaved the other side of his head; and no longer did he sprint out into the streets barefoot. He occasionally talked about Jesus and being an assistant district attorney, but rarely, and with a fraction of the former fervor. One day he stopped carrying around the legal pads altogether.

All settings have their model citizens—the exemplars of propriety—and from the time the Haldol trickled through his synapses, Rex became the poster boy of the shelter. He was cordial, abstemious, and gracious. He cofacilitated groups on the dangers of substance abuse. He grew physically healthier and put on a bit of much-needed weight. The hollowed-out crack look in his face receded and was replaced by a sanguine glow. Within a few months he was declared by José and the staff to be "housing ready." Rex moved out of the Barracks and into a brand-new, gleaming, supportive housing residence, where I was helping conduct research and where he had his own apartment, with kitchen, bedroom, and living room in a gentrifying area of New Haven. To facilitate the transition, Rex was visited weekly in his new residence by José, who offered support, gauged how the adjustment to more independent living was going, and served as an advocate for Rex and liaison to me and the other residential staff. José's efforts were part of a planned intervention and research study in which clients leaving the shelters were randomly assigned to one of two groups. One group received no follow-up from the shelter staff after they left the shelter (they received the "usual care," which meant a handshake and the conferring of best wishes); the second group, of which Rex was a part, received nine months of follow-up care to ease and facilitate the transition out of the shelter and into supportive housing.

Rex adjusted wonderfully to his new place of residence. He took his medications and abstained from crack. He was voted by his peers to be a client representative to staff. He got a part-time minimum-wage job as a messenger. He kept his new apartment immaculately clean. He set the dining table for five extra places—two for his parents, one for his sister, one for his daughter, and one for his granddaughter. (In the intervening months, Rex, at age thirty-two, became a grandfather, after his sixteen-year-old daughter had a baby with an indeterminate father.) His family, who lived in Boston and had many problems of their own, never appeared at the table, but Rex liked the feeling of being ready for them should they ever show up. While not as viscerally dramatic and rapid a transformation as depicted in the Oliver Sacks–inspired movie *Awakenings*, Rex's metamorphosis was just as profound. He fully reengaged and reentered the world. Rex was living a new life of grace, and the only remnants of his former self were his boom box and the fact that his clothes were slightly more lurid than would be considered normal. The entire transition had occurred in less than two years.

And Rex did become an assistant district attorney, after a fashion. A letter arrived summoning Rex for jury duty. Putting on his best suit, he reported to the court off the New Haven Green and returned to the residence reporting that he had been selected for service. As the director of the residence, I wondered if I should intervene. I decided, in consultation with others, that Rex's medical history was a private matter and that the legal system should be free to make up its mind about what responsibilities to assign him. When Rex came back a few days later to report that he had been named jury captain, I wondered if that was such a good idea. Still, the staff and I remained discreet, and Rex happily went to court to captain his jury daily for about two months. Whatever the trial was about, it must have been very serious. We never found out, as Rex dutifully never revealed a bit of information about the proceedings. One day Rex simply announced that the trial was over and that he had discharged his duties. For a considerable time afterwards, he carried himself with a resolute, unbending, and powerful sense of pride.

The researchers completed their study. They found that, in the eighteen-month period after clients left the shelter, the group who received nine months of transitional follow-up care was dramatically less likely to reexperience homelessness than those who had no transitional support. Those who received no follow-up were homeless for an average of ninety days during that eighteen-month period, while those with nine-month follow-up were homeless for an average of thirty days. In the world of research, which is far murkier and more mysterious than outsiders might think, this is a decisive finding. It showed that for people with mental illness and a chronic history of homelessness, a thoughtful aftercare program could break a recurrent pattern of returning to the streets.[35]

A few years later, the same team of researchers looked at the data in a different way. The symptoms of schizophrenia are generally divided into two categories, positive and negative. Positive symptoms refer to the active psychotic symptoms such as hallucinations (hearing voices, seeing things that other people don't see) and delusions (having distorted beliefs, typically of a paranoid nature). Negative symptoms are "quieter" but just as debilitating and include social withdrawal, poor hygiene, lack of motivation, emotional flattening, and inability to experience pleasure—that quality of being cut off from the rest of the world, and even from themselves, that characterizes so many people with the illness. While positive symptoms get the newspaper headlines, negative symptoms are in many ways more debilitating and certainly harder to treat. (Medications can do a good job with the voices and the delusions, but they don't usually alleviate the negative symptoms, and sometimes they make them worse.) It is an extraordinarily difficult clinical challenge to get people who suffer from schizophrenia to be reengaged with themselves and with the world. Using a scale that measures positive and negative symptoms, the researchers assessed the two groups. The nine-month-follow-up group, in addition to having two-thirds less homelessness, had a statistically significant decrease in negative symptoms. So it wasn't just Rex; collectively the men had started to come out of their shells. Given the intractable nature of negative symptoms, this finding has potentially important clinical significance.

Neuroimaging has shown that negative symptoms are associated with problems in the prefrontal cortex of the brain. The authors of the study conclude: "One intriguing possibility is that by encouraging patients to focus on . . . their transition from institution to community living, the Critical Time Intervention provides cognitive remediation, helping to reactivate prefrontal cortical functions as they are summoned to carry out executive [decision-making] tasks that were underutilized during lengthy periods of passivity and regression [in institutional care]."[36]

John Curtis, a psychologist and expert on the neurobiology of resilience (which he defines as good adaptation in the face of adverse events) at the University of Rochester, explained to me what might have transpired in Rex's brain. "There's no doubt that there were chemical and structural changes that occurred in Rex's brain as a result of some of the positive things that he was exposed to when he got off crack and into treatment. The chemical changes were introduced by the Haldol, which clearly worked beautifully for him. You could say that the Haldol was a critical event, one that created the scaffolding, if you will, for the other changes to occur. It made his brain plastic enough to be ready to change when he was exposed to better things in the environment. But just as profoundly, the enriched environment that he experienced when he moved into housing—the support from José, the better food, sleeping eight hours a night, social stimulation, having supportive role models—all changed his brain, too. One can think of it as a bidirectional, or dialectical flow, between the drug and the environment. Together, it can have an additive effect."

"But how would you describe what might have been going on in his brain?" I ask.

"Well, this is all speculative, but most likely anatomically, his prefrontal cortex changed. He was making new axons and dendrites. The size of his neurons could have been changing. Certainly new synaptic connections were being forged, causing a reworking and rewiring of the brain based on positive experience."

And so in Rex's story, social neuroscience comes full circle: social engagement, treatment engagement, diet, medication, emphasis on strengths and respect for personal autonomy, changes in the brain, and recovery in the context of illness.

I am reminded of the plot of one of the adventures of Tintin, the French cartoon character who goes on adventures around the world. In *The Secret of the Unicorn*, and its sequel, *Red Rackham's Treasure*, Tintin and his friend Captain Haddock undertake a massive and perilous journey to South America to find buried treasure. It turns out that the treasure all along had been in the basement of Marlinspike, their home in France. They just didn't know it was there.

Postscript

Emotional Rescue

If anyone was ever genetically loaded for suicidal behavior, it was Walker Percy, who so wisely predicted the ascendance of Corporate Psychiatry and the Prozac-in-the-water phenomenon.

"Melancholy and suicide have a prominent place in the Percy family saga," wrote Walker's biographer.[1] The first Percy to arrive in America, Charles, tied a sugar kettle to his neck, strolled into a Mississippi creek at the end of January, and drowned himself in 1794. Walker's paternal grandfather committed suicide with a twelve-gauge shotgun in 1917. His father, a brilliant and successful lawyer who suffered from deep depression and insomnia, did the same twelve years later with a twenty-gauge. Two years after his father's suicide, Percy's mother drowned when her car ran off a bridge not far from their home. It may have been intentional. Walker and his brothers were taken in by their enigmatic and well-educated "Uncle Will," their father's cousin, who was a lawyer and author. Walker adored Uncle Will and said that he saved his life. If it hadn't been for Uncle Will, Percy once said, he probably would have ended up a car dealer in Athens, Georgia.[2] Percy said later that he had spent his entire life and work trying to answer a single question: "Why did my father kill himself?"[3]

Walker went to college at the University of North Carolina and studied chemistry. Influenced by Julian Huxley and H. G. Wells, he put his faith in science, believing for a time in his life that it was capable of solving all the world's mysteries and miseries. After completing medical school at Columbia, Percy contracted tuberculosis while performing autopsies at Bellevue Hospital. Bedridden for the next three years, he was exhausted and often depressed; he spent much time reading works of the existentialists Camus, Sartre, and Kierkegaard, as well as the writings of Catholic thinkers Blaise Pascal, Romano Guardini, and St. Thomas Aquinas. These writers allowed him to question the scientific, materialist view of reality. Years later Percy wrote, "What did at last dawn on me as a medical student and intern, a practitioner, I thought, of the scientific method, was that there was a huge gap in the scientific view of the world. This sector of the world about which science could not utter a single word was nothing less than this: what it is like to be an individual living in the United States in the twentieth century."[4] In his odd but brilliant 1983 satire *Lost in the Cosmos: The Last Self-Help Book*, Percy combines an analysis of the ills of our age with some tentative suggestions about what do about them. *Lost in the Cosmos* is a departure for Percy in that instead of a novel, it is a sort of memorandum to his fellow wayfarers in American society. This is pure and unvarnished Percy, relieved of the need to tell a story. For the reader, this is liberating, because narrative was not his primary gift.

Throughout the book, Percy plays with the concept of "reentry." There are two types of souls, according to Percy: those with their feet firmly on the ground and in tune with the world, and those other people, those sensitive souls who are out of sorts with the world, "out of the here-and-now." Percy (whose writing often verged on science fiction) says these people are orbiting the world, rather than being fully part of it. Many of these struggling people are trying to figure out various forms of what Percy calls reentry. By reentry, Percy means various methods of getting through life, or as he says "how to get through a Wednesday afternoon." (Or as the Irish rock band the Pogues sing:

"Too many sad days, Too many Tuesday mornings.") Percy was writing explicitly about writers and artists, who have made a tradition of having reentry difficulties, but Percy makes clear that his reentry stratagems apply to everyone bothered by their current circumstances in the world; in other words, the many depressed, troubled, sensitive people who are having problems trying to come to terms with the world. In other words, those who are in an unwelcome and intrusive amount of pain. In other words, Julie in Winterset.

Based on the life histories of various historical figures, Percy devises the following list of well-trodden attempts at reentry, both successful and unsuccessful. Some of the people used as examples are Percy's; some are mine:

> *Reentry, uneventful and self intact:* This would be Walker Percy's equivalent of "the healthy-minded." This, Percy points out, is exceedingly rare.

> *Reentry by anesthesia:* That is, drugs and alcohol, or, as Percy puts it, rendering "the intolerable tolerable by a chemical assault on the cortex of the brain." Shining examples: F. Scott Fitzgerald, Brendan Behan, Dylan Thomas, Keith Richards.

> *Reentry through travel (geographical):* Relentless moving from place to place in order to distract oneself from oneself. Examples: D. H. Lawrence, Ernest Hemingway, Graham Greene, Jack Kerouac, Bob Dylan.

> *Reentry by travel (sexual):* Taking on a succession of lovers. Examples: D. H. Lawrence, Henry Miller, Anaïs Nin, Robert Mapplethorpe, Madonna.

> *Reentry by return:* Returning to the place one left, as a way of controlling and understanding one's origin and one's life. Examples: None. Percy says, "You can't go home again."

Reentry by disguise: The aping of people who have successfully reentered the world. In other words, trying to be healthy-minded when you're not.

Reentry by Eastern window: The adoption of Hinduism, Buddhism, Zen, the Moonies, et cetera. Examples: Aldous Huxley, Christopher Isherwood, George Harrison.

Reentry under the direct sponsorship of God: Dietrich Bonhoeffer, Thomas Merton (and Percy himself, who converted to Catholicism in his thirties and embraced it devoutly for the rest of his life).

Reentry deferred, or self indefinitely withdrawn into orbit: J. D. Salinger in the woods, Proust in his bed.

Refusal of reentry and exit into deep space (i.e., suicide): Virginia Woolf, Ernest Hemingway, Spalding Gray, at one point, almost, Percy himself.

If one were to employ Percy's concepts and bring them to bear on the last fifteen years of American history, one would have to say that the sick souls of Americans have gone in a little heavily for one particular method of getting to the second story. And that would be: REENTRY BY ANTIDEPRESSANTS.

Or as the pharmaceutical companies would no doubt prefer to put it: REENTRY BY SELECTIVE SEROTONIN REUPTAKE INHIBITION.

This has been the reentry path most favored and cherished by our Julie. This has certainly been the mode of reentry favored by the American public, and like Percy's other modes of reentry, reentry by antidepressants has both a history of success and a history of failure. We now know the numerous problems with an overreliance on antidepressants as a reentry mode for sick souls, and, as we have seen, in concentrating so relentlessly on a single form of reentry, by antidepressants, we have tragically overlooked other forms of reentry, which are often more effective:

Reentry by realizing there are no panaceas for emotional ills
Reentry by psychotherapy
And more specifically, reentry by cognitive-behavioral therapy
Reentry by exercise
Reentry by fish oil
Reentry by someone who helped me find my own motivation to change
Reentry by using one's strengths
Reentry by social engagement
Reentry by finding a reason to live
Reentry by recovery—finding ways to live a productive life even in the midst of ongoing and painful symptoms
Reentry by being the expert in one's self.

I have three modest proposals for alternate forms of Reentry by Antidepressants, or by Serotonin Reuptake. Please note that these are not clinical paths. These are not scientific ideas and will not be subjected—indeed, could not be subjected—to any randomized clinical trials. I can readily attest that these ideas will not be published in a professional journal anytime soon. But here are some suggestions of some new ways of looking at things:

ALTERNATE STRATEGY NUMBER ONE: Reentry by the Healthiness and Sanity of Depression

Healthiness of Depression? How could that be?

Yes, I would argue that depression (small *d*) can be good. Let me explain.

As in the discussion about Julie, I am talking here about depression, and not Depression. I am not talking here about the suffering of schizophrenia, of bipolar disorder, of major depression. I am making the distinction, as I have throughout this narrative, between people with severe psychiatric pathology and those who are simply bothered by things. The suffering and horror of delusions and hallucinations of schizophrenia, the horrendous mood swings of bipolar disorder, the desperate torpor of major depression, the misery of eating disorders—all that true medical ill health—need to be redressed and controlled. While a cure is unlikely, mental illness can be managed so that people can lead tolerable and productive existences. But I would contend that depression, in the sense of feeling things—feeling sad, feeling upset, feeling bothered—in these times is a good thing and an appropriate response. Look at the headlines: car bombs in Iraq; teenage girls killed by predators they encounter on myspace .com; lying presidents; melting snows in the Antarctic; corporate scandals, not to mention the old staples of death, mortality, and disease. Maybe, if you feel sadness at such things, you're aware and sensitive and alive. Maybe it's a credit to your constitution, demonstrating that you are capable of thinking, feeling, responding, breathing, and yes, suffering.

As Percy says in *Lost in the Cosmos:*

> Assume that you are quite right [to be depressed]. You are depressed because you have every reason to be depressed. No member of the other two million species which inhabit the earth—and who are luckily exempt from depression—would fail to be depressed if it lived the life you lead. You live in a deranged age—more deranged than usual, because despite great scientific and technological advances, man has not the faintest idea of who he is or what he is doing . . . Consider the only adults who are never depressed: chuckleheads, California surfers, and fundamentalist Christians who believe they have had a personal encounter with Jesus and are saved for once and all.[5]

Percy's comments bring to mind the scene in *Annie Hall* when Alvy Singer, played by Woody Allen, struggling with the difficulties of being in this world, encounters a handsome, untroubled-looking couple—

blond, peppy, and preppy, with beautiful teeth and shiny hair—on the street:

"You look like a very happy couple—um, are you?" Alvy asks.

The man answers, "Yeah."

"So, so how do you account for it?"

The man says, "Well, I'm very shallow and empty, and I have no ideas and nothing interesting to say." The unblemished girl adds brightly, "And I'm exactly the same way."

Woody says, "I see! Wow! That's very interesting. So you've managed to work out something?"

They nod happily.

A certain measure of depression is absolutely appropriate to this world. Indeed, it can be a sign of health, an indicator of being a thinking, feeling person—proof that one is alive. It is this line of reasoning that James Agee, a feeling soul himself, explored in *Let Us Now Praise Famous Men* when he wrote, "As a whole part of 'psychological education' it needs to be remembered that a neurosis can be valuable; also that 'adjustment' to a sick and insane environment is of itself not health but sickness and insanity."

There is also, of course, an evolutionary usefulness to many "bad" emotions. Martin Seligman phrased it succinctly in an interview a few years ago: "Anxiety, depression, and anger have long evolutionary histories in which they're trying to tell us something. Depression, feeling sad, tells us we've lost something. Anger alerts us to trespass, anxiety alerts us to danger. Insofar as we jump in and try and dampen the alarm system, we do so at our peril." These indicators are not fail-safe alarm systems: we have a tendency to overreact, to be sure, but at their fundaments, these signaling systems are good and useful things. They are messages that we need to hear. They give us vital feedback on our progress, or lack of it, through our interior and exterior environment or, as Seligman put it, negative emotions contain "messages about how our commerce with the world is going."[6]

Other cultures know that emotional pain is a good thing. In Japanese culture, for instance, sadness is appropriate and valued. "Melancholia, sensitivity, fragility—these are not negative things in a Japanese context," Tohru Takahashi, a psychiatrist who worked for Japan's National Institute of Mental Health for three decades, explained. "It never occurred to us that we should try to remove [sad and melancholy emotions], because it never occurred to us that they were bad."[7] Hayao Kawai, a clinical psychologist who became Japan's commissioner of cultural affairs, said, "Nature shows us that life is sadness, that everything dies or ends . . . Our mythology repeats that; we do not have stories where anyone lives happily ever after."[8]

Because depression was not considered a negative condition, SSRIs have been slow to take hold in Japan. No SSRIs were sold there until 1999. In order to create a market, pharmaceutical companies had to actually invent a phrase for mild depression: *kokoro no kaze*, which, roughly translated, means one's soul catching cold. After furnishing the catchy phrase, the drug companies followed up with all the usual artillery that had worked so well in the West: public awareness campaigns paid for by the drug companies and an army of 1,350 Paxil representatives who canvassed selected doctors an average of twice a week. As a result, visits to doctors for depression in Japan went up 46 percent between 1999 to 2003, and sales of anti-depressants increased 500 percent during that time. When asked why GlaxoSmithKline went ahead with campaigns promoting depression and antidepressants, the Japanese product manager for Paxil explained: "When other pharmaceutical companies were giving up on developing antidepressants in Japan, we went ahead for a very simple reason: the successful marketing in the United States and Europe."[9]

In America, we have too long been held prisoner to the sentiment expressed in that most American of songs, "Over the Rainbow"—that someday, somewhere, somehow, magically and inexorably, all will be bliss, that our troubles will melt like "lemon drops" and that dreams really do come true.

Hollywood, it's time for a rewrite.

. . .

My second modest suggestion:

ALTERNATE STRATEGY NUMBER TWO: Reentry by Emotional Contrasts

We would be nowhere without some emotional pain. Life is best lived with contrast. Pain and pleasure are indelibly linked, and I believe that some of the richest soaring peaks of happiness are a direct product of having difficult times. I have long believed that relief—which is no more than the ending of pain or anxiety—is one of the most exquisite emotions imaginable. The elation of finding an important document that one believed had been lost, the sheer sense of physical well-being after surviving a nasty bout with the flu, the quiet of recovery after a traumatic incident, the peace after the storm . . . In my work with the homeless, among the most downtrodden and desperate members of society, I found that there were constant moments of humor and levity even in the midst of gloom.

What follows is a passage from *A Portrait of the Artist as a Young Man* by James Joyce. This is Stephen Dedalus after he has confessed to a priest about being with a prostitute:

> He knelt to say his penance, praying in a corner of the dark nave; and his prayers ascended to heaven from his purified heart like perfume streaming upwards from a heart of white rose.
>
> The muddy streets were gay. He strode homeward, conscious of an invisible grace pervading and making light his limbs. In spite of all he had done it. He had confessed and God had pardoned him. His soul was made fair and holy once more, holy and happy . . .
>
> He sat by the fire in the kitchen, not daring to speak for happiness. Till that moment he had not known how beautiful and peaceful life could be. The green square of paper pinned round the lamp cast down a tender shade. On the dresser was a plate of sausages and white pudding and on the shelf there were eggs. They would be for the breakfast in the morning after the

> communion in the college chapel. White pudding and eggs and sausages and cups of tea. How simple and beautiful was life after all! And life lay all before him.[10]

Without the anguish, the simple and pure beauty would not have happened.

The second point is that difficult times, stress, and friction very often lead to achievement. Michael Jordan couldn't make his high school basketball team. Arguably the greatest Anglo-American leaders of the nineteenth and twentieth centuries—Lincoln and Churchill—suffered from depression. Nelson Mandela came out of prison, as did Malcolm X; Martin Luther King Jr. rose out of the oppression of the South. Most great entertainers, writers, songwriters, thinkers spend a good deal of time on the margins before they come up with anything interesting. When Walker Percy was asked why so much great literature came out of the American South, he said: "Simple, we lost."

It's like Orson Welles, playing the villain Harry Lime in the classic British movie *The Third Man.* Welles is confronted by his former friend, played by Joseph Cotten, about his bad behavior, which in this case is selling penicillin on the black market. The dramatic, conclusive confrontation occurs on Vienna's Riesenrad, a massive Ferris wheel. With the Austrian capital's skyline behind him and the Danube River and the Vienna Woods below, Harry Lime justifies his behavior and the conflicts he has created: "In Italy for thirty years under the Borgias they had warfare, terror, murder, bloodshed—and they produced Michelangelo, Leonardo da Vinci, and the Renaissance. In Switzerland, they had brotherly love—five hundred years of democracy and peace. And what did that produce? The cuckoo clock."

Let's call it not the Sea Snail syndrome but the Steve Earle syndrome, referring to the extremely talented singer-songwriter who produced only middling material early in his career, with a few frustratingly brief flashes of brilliance, until both his career and his health dwindled as a result of being caught in a vortex of cocaine, crack, and alcohol. With a five-hundred-dollar-a-day habit, Earle pawned his guitars and became homeless. His most gainful employment for a time was as a doorman of an after-hours crack house. Earle eventually went to prison for two years, where he was not allowed either a guitar or pen. Since his release from prison, he has produced a torrent of soulful, stunning albums, a book of short stories, a play; he has also formed his own record label, produced many records by other artists, taught music, and become a stalwart and active opponent of the death penalty. He's won a Grammy and been called by *Esquire* "the finest narrative songwriter around."[11] All of that in about ten years. "I didn't write anything for four and a half years at the end of my drug use, so you know, it's amazing how much energy you suddenly have when you don't have to wake up in the morning and score five hundred dollars' worth of dope. I think it makes you look at everything a little differently, makes you do everything a lot differently. So I don't waste much energy or time now . . . I'm disgustingly happy right now."[12]

We don't need to seek it out, but when it descends, it's important to make good use of our pain. As Rainer Maria Rilke wrote in *The Duino Elegies:*

> How we squander our hours of pain. How we gaze beyond them into the bitter duration to see if they have an end. Though they are really our winter-enduring foliage, our dark evergreen, one season in our inner year—not only a season in time—but are place and settlement, foundation and soil and home.[13]

Instead, we've embarked on a uniquely American process of emotional sanitation. We have been equally driven to inoculate ourselves against the rough-and-tumble aspects of existence. But death, pain, strife are the constants. Look at the great stories, the great teachers, the great writers: the Bible, the Koran, Shakespeare, Dante, Melville, Dostoevsky, Tolstoy, Dickens, Emily Dickinson, the films of Hitchcock and Scorsese. All of these stories are absolutely dense with turmoil and murder, hell and high water, fear and loathing. The fact is that those things, rather than numbed-out emotions, have characterized most of humanity's tenure on earth, and always will.

And finally,

ALTERNATE STRATEGY NUMBER THREE: Reentry by Mystery

One last possibility needs to be raised. It's just possible that we will never figure out and remedy our psychiatric suffering. It is just conceivable that psychiatric illness is just so complicated that we will always suffer from ongoing depression and anxiety. What ails Julie will never be cured. Kate George, an analyst at IMS Health, the leading research group of the drug industry, wrote soberly: "Depression is a genetically complex disorder . . . and behavior is complex and multifactorial." This complexity, she added, "combined with the infancy of these biotech programs, means that a groundbreaking pharmacologic therapy or use of tailored therapy for depression is a long way off—and may never be possible at all."[14]

I am sometimes oddly, perhaps perversely, comforted by the limits of what we can know, measure, and predict. No matter how much progress neuroscience makes, there will always be something that remains ineffably mysterious and unknowable about ourselves. Science is still mainly filled with the unknown. The unknown is greater than the known. We are destined to be forever blind voyagers and fellow wayfarers.

But rather than condemn ourselves for how little we know, or worse, pump up and inflate the value of the paltry state of our current knowledge, perhaps it is better simply to accept these limitations. In our flaws and in our ignorance, there is mystery. And mystery is what makes us human and complicated and interesting. There is and always will be something enduringly inscrutable about humanity, and therein lies the beauty.

As Glen Gabbard, the psychiatrist at Baylor, said to me, there will always be two languages: the language of neuroscience—the language of neurotransmitters, synapses, neurons, brain imaging; and the language of human experience—thoughts, ideas, feelings, object relations.[15] No matter how much progress biological psychiatry makes, the two languages will never meet. There will never be a one-to-one correspondence between neuroscience and lived experience. The best diagnostic tool in psychiatry is still simply to ask the patient what he feels. If machines tell us otherwise, who are we going to believe, the patient or the machine? The day that we choose the machine's word over a person's, we have lost the game. Won the battle but lost the war.

It is like trying to capture a snowflake: it melts the moment you catch it. There remains, in my opinion, something ineffably and permanently unknowable about the human predicament—unpredictable, wonderful, horrible, not easily or ever reducible to being a "pack of neurons."

It's okay. Our salvation is in our mystery. Our mystery is in our salvation. It is what makes us interesting.

Psychiatry, after all, is charged with the hardest questions in medicine.

What makes us suffer?
What makes us better?
How do we change?

Getting at those answers is nigh impossible. As Nietzsche said: "We are unknown, we knowers, to ourselves." Or as one of the world's most influential neuroscientists, confided to me, with his guard down: "The brain, it's just really, really complicated."

I recall a psychiatrist, Dr. Anthony Roper, telling me sometime in the mid-1990s, in the heady days of Prozac Nation and the rapid-fire construction of the Serotonin Empire, that patients should take the least amount of psychiatric medications that they need. "I believe you take the minimal amount of medication you can," he said. At the time, amid high hopes for all the new drugs, and an insularity to their side effects and various consequences, this advice sounded old-fashioned, odd, even a little radical. As straightforward and sensible as Dr. Roper's statement was, his was a lonely belief indeed at the time he made it.

In retrospect, Dr. Roper's pronouncement is timeless. Of course, we should take the least amount of drugs that we can! It's a law that applies to cold medicine, antibiotics, and interferon, as well as antidepressants and antipsychotics.

Take what you need, when you need it, and judiciously set the rest aside. Respect the power and complexity, as well as the limitations, of the drugs. And I would add, as Dr. Roper was saying: Take the least amount of the drugs you need, and maximize other, human ways to solve problems.

If there's any lesson to be gleaned from the recent history of psychiatry, it is, in T. M. Luhrmann's words, "how complex mental illness is, how difficult it is to treat, and how, in the face of this complexity, people cling to coherent explanations like poor swimmers to a raft."[16] Psychopharmacological overenthusiasm—as evidenced by the habits of the citizens of Winterset, Iowa, and the rest of the United States—is simply the latest of these overreactions, just as psychoanalysis was once thought capable of curing the ills of society and behaviorism of creating utopian communities. Given the complexity of our problems, we can ill afford to jettison one approach or the other.

We have arrived at a particular and potentially decisive moment in the brief but highly eventful history of psychopharmacological overenthusiasm. We don't know much, but we should know just enough to recognize how primitive and crude our understanding of psychiatric drugs are.

Which way will we go for our emotional rescue? Which way will we turn? Will we continue our reckless ingesting of drugs, our simplistic explanations of human behavior?

Or will we, with an open mind, heed the lessons from a century of research on psychotherapy and motivation and what enhances people's prospects for change? Will we accept that illness and suffering are part of humanity, and that understanding that only helps us to overcome that suffering? Will we comprehend that change comes slowly and through hard work?

Will we accept, in humility, that the ills of this world have a tantalizing way of eluding simple explanation? Will we see that progress, when it comes, usually comes slowly, contrary to our preference?

Our only hope is to be resolute and careful, not faddish, in assessing new developments as they arise and adopting them judiciously within a tradition of a gradually but steadily growing armamentarium in the fight against genuine human suffering.

Acknowledgments

I would first like to thank Betsy Lerner, my agent, who is so much more than an agent. As in: editor, erstwhile therapist, friend. Among many other contributions, Betsy helped me formulate the proposal for this book and guided me expertly and kindly through the emotional highs and lows of the entire process. I count myself lucky to be working with her.

Similar sentiments can be expressed to Dan Frank, editorial director at Pantheon, and his colleague Fran Bigman. Dan's perspicacity in seeing the forest for the trees improved this book profoundly. He has always been kind, patient, and supportive. Fran's stamp is all over this book—I am exceedingly grateful to her for keeping me "on track," and, under Dan's guidance, for providing me with some absolutely critical editorial advice. Fran also has been unceasingly gracious and forever helpful. She has a brilliant career ahead of her as an editor. I would also like to thank the many people at Pantheon and Random House who help make a book, in particular Katie Freeman, Janice Goldklang, Elizabeth Calamari, Anke Steinecke, Soonyoung Kwon, Peter Mendelsund and the extraordinarily patient and meticulous Victoria Pearson. I am appreciative, as well, of the careful work by proofreaders Carol Rutan and Judy Eda.

I would like to thank the many scientists, clinicians, and industry analysts who I talked to, interviewed, and consulted with. I was astonished at how responsive and helpful the following were to my inquiries: Steven Arnold, Helen Bach-Mizrachi, Stephen Bank, Judith Beck,

Roger Blashfield, Heather Cameron, John Curtis, Larry Davidson, Carlo DiClemente, Kathryn Dudley, Ronald Duman, Robert Ehrlich, Amelia Eisch, Alan Felix, Lisa Fenton, Thomas Fuchs, Glen Gabbard, Paul Gordon, Richard Gordon, Marc Gourevitch, Charles Gross, Ronald Gurrera, Matthew Herper, Kim Hopper, Eric Kandel, Joan Kaufman, Jerald Kay, John Laub, Jerry Lowenstein, Tanya Luhrmann, Angus MacDonald, John Mack, Scott Masters, Bill Miller, Mike Miller, Terry Moyers, Kim Mueser, Siddharta Nadkarni, Mike Neale, Eric Nestler, Mark Olfson, Lewis Opler, Christopher Pittenger, Robyn Redinger, Robert Sampson, Gerard Sanacora, Mark Senak, Edward Shorter, John Strauss, Elliot Valenstein, Bill Vaughan, Myrna Weissman, and Henny Westra. A number of scientists and practitioners were especially helpful, responding to repeated questions, or reading and commenting on extended passages. They are Gloster Aaron, Victoria Arango, Hal Arkowitz, Lisa Fenton, Michele Klimczak, and Gerard Sanacora. I would also like to thank Jordan Besek for some timely research assistance.

I am especially grateful to David Healy for being so consistently helpful and generous in sharing his remarkable knowledge base about the history of psychopharmacology with me. Michael Rowe read drafts and provided comments in his characteristically modest yet brilliant manner. I think I incorporated every suggestion he made. Another mentor, Richard Ohmann, scrupulously read and commented on the manuscript and always, always, got to the heart of the matter. Other writers have helped me considerably over the years: among them, Lis Harris, Jonathan Schell, William Finnegan, and Jennifer Gonnerman (who has been absolutely extraordinary in her support of this project). Anne Greene, director of the Wesleyan Writers Program, has been instrumental in my career (as she has been with so many writers) and hired me to teach at Wesleyan in the middle of this book's genesis. I am appreciative of two writers for whom I worked as a young man and who influenced me greatly: William Manchester and Paul Horgan. And also to Robert Coles: my model of what it is to be a writer-practitioner-teacher.

Thanks to all members of the Yale Psychiatry and Psychology writers group who tolerated my reading early drafts of this book over many years—Mike Neale, David Sells, John Strauss, Raquel Andres-Hyman, Elizabeth Flanagan, Heather Goff. And thank you to friends who kept me going with their cheers: Alex Bloom, Robin Fox, Jason Gold, Amy Kalafa, David Marchetti, and Corinne Thurstan.

The Yale Program for Recovery and Community Health provided ongoing support: in particular, its directors, Larry Davidson and the aforementioned Michael Rowe. They are prolific researchers and greatly influenced my understanding of the "recovery" issues discussed in this book.

I owe a special thanks to people at The Connection, an extraordinarily innovative social services agency with programs throughout Connecticut that in so many ways has become my home in recent years—and where many of the ideas explored in the second half of this book are being tested and implemented, to excellent effect. Specifically I am in debt to Peter Nucci, The Connection's CEO, who has understood my idiosyncratic ways and blessed me with remarkable freedom; to Pat Clark, who good naturedly read everything I wrote and explored issues with me from her knowledgeable and wise perspective; and to David D'Amora, for his challenging and inspirational edge and enormous expertise. For technical assistance and humor, I thank Scott Morris. For their consistent warmth and support, I also thank Heide Erb, Lynn Spencer, and Lisa DeMatteis.

My father, by diligent example, showed me how to write and research—or "dig," as he would put it—even if it meant getting up at two in the morning to write down an idea before it disappeared. My mother provided a literary model and made me want to become a writer. My brothers Tom and John—writers both—read the manuscript with the appropriate mixture of enthusiasm and incisive critique, and of love and support.

Writing a book involves being in a relationship with a computer screen for nights, months, years at a time. For understanding that, tolerating that, and even encouraging that, I deeply thank my wife,

Laura, and son, Louis. Laura and Louis, too, know how to get to the essence of things, and they pushed me and steadied me at all the right times. For putting up with my long absences, my memory lapses, and my distracted air for years at a time, I owe a debt beyond words.

Notes

FOREWORD: "SO HIP, SO QUICKLY"

1. Ceci Connolly, "Tipper Gore Details Depression Treatment," *The Washington Post,* May 8, 1999.
2. The White House, Office of the Press Secretary, "President Says U.S. Must Make Commitment to Mental Health Care," press conference, April 29, 2002, www.whitehouse.gov/news/releases/2002/04/20020429-1.html, accessed August 23, 2007.
3. Lance S. Longwell, senior manager, Public Relations, IMS Health, personal correspondence, June 15, 2007.
4. Ibid.
5. M. N. Stagnitti, "Trends in Antidepressant Use by the U.S. Civilian Noninstitutionalized Population, 1997 and 2002," Statistical Brief #76, May 2005, Agency for Healthcare Research and Quality, Rockville, MD.
6. Margaret L. Eaton, "Developing and Marketing a Blockbuster Drug: Lessons from Eli Lilly's Experience with Prozac," Case Study: Stanford Graduate School of Business, February 25, 2005.
7. M. Olfson, S. C. Marcus, M. Tedeschi, and G. J. Wan, "Continuity of Antidepressant Treatment for Adults with Depression in the United States," *American Journal of Psychiatry* 163 (January 2006): 101–108.
8. Top 10 Therapeutic Classes by U.S. Dispensed Prescriptions, IMS Health, March 2007.

9. S. J. Rupke, D. Blecke, and M. Renfrow, "Cognitive Therapy for Depression," *American Family Physician*, vol. 73, no. 1, January 1, 2006. G. A. Fava, C. Rafanelli, S. Grandi, and S. Conti, "Prevention of Recurrent Depression with Cognitive Behavioral Therapy," *Archives of General Psychiatry*, vol. 55, 1998, 816–20.
10. N. A. Landenberg and M. W. Lipsey, "The Positive Effects of Cognitive-Behavioral Programs for Offenders: A Meta-Analysis of Factors Associated with Effective Treatment," *Journal of Experimental Criminology*, 1, no. 4 (December 2005).
11. Scott Allen, "Antidepressants' Risk of Suicide Now Called Low," *Boston Globe*, January 1, 2006.
12. National Institute of Mental Health. Questions and Answers About the NIMH Clinical Antipsychotic Trials of Intervention Effectiveness Study (CATIE)—Phase 2 Results, April 1, 2006.
13. American Psychiatric Association, "Landmark STAR*D Depression Study Offers Sobering Third-Round Results," news release, July 1, 2006.

CHAPTER ONE: WHO MEDICATED IOWA?

1. *Winterset Madisonian*, March 21, 2007.
2. www.gowinteret.com, accessed August 20, 2007.
3. *Madison County Agriculture*, prepared by Daniel Otto, Iowa State University, University Extension, November 2006, http://www.extension.iastate.edu/Publications/PM202-61.pdf, accessed August 20, 2007.
4. http://www.reagan.utexas.edu/archives/speeches/1984/110384d.htm, accessed August 20, 2007.
5. "Convenience Store Robbed," *Winterset Madisonian*, August 23, 2006. "Public a No-Show at City Budget Hearing," *Winterset Madisonian*, March 7, 2007.
6. The Wellmark Report, Seventh in a Series of Special Reports: Antidepressants, http://www.wellmark.com/health_improvement/reports/charts/antidepressants/antidepressants_IA.htm, accessed August 23, 2007.
7. Yahoo! Answers, "Does Paxil Numb Your Emotions?" http://answers

.yahoo.com/question/index?qid=20070528165631AABz4Qf, accessed June 10, 2007.

8. Malcolm Gladwell, "Big and Bad," *The New Yorker*, January 12, 2004. Ben Greenman. Q&A: Roadkillers. Interview with Malcolm Gladwell. *The New Yorker* online. January 12, 2004. www.thenewyorker.com/archive/2004/01/12/040112on_onlineonly01, accessed September 23, 2007.
9. David Healy, *Let Them Eat Prozac* (New York and London: New York University Press, 2004), p. 39.
10. Eaton, "Developing and Marketing a Blockbuster Drug."
11. Patricia Filip, "OSU's 2003 Alumni Fellows: Prozac Co-Discoverer David Wong," *Oregon Stater*, December 2003, http://alumni.oregonstate.edu/stater/issues/stater0312/alumnifellows.html, accessed July 31, 2007.
12. T. M. Luhrmann, *Of Two Minds: An Anthropologist Looks at American Psychiatry* (New York: Vintage Books, 2000), p. 211.
13. United Press International, "Study: Psych Drugs Sales Up," March 28, 2007, www.upi.com/Health_Business, accessed September 20, 2007.
14. United Press International, 1997 stats are: "Study: Psych Drugs Sales Up," 2006 (IMS) stats are: IMS Health, Top 10 Therapeutic Classes by U.S. Sales, www.imshealth.org, accessed May 13, 2007.
15. Wolter Kluwer Health, "Estimated Unique Patient Counts, May 2007," www.lexapro.com/about_lexapro/what_is.aspx, accessed August 28, 2007.
16. Gallup Poll, "How Many Teens Are on Mood Medication?" February 22, 2005, www.galluppoll.com, accessed April 9, 2007.
17. Jonathan Mahler, "The Antidepressant Dilemma," *The New York Times Magazine*, November 21, 2004.
18. Carla Hall, "Pets Join 'Prozac Nation,' " *Los Angeles Times*, January 16, 2007.
19. IMS Health, "Antidepressants—Total U.S. Sales $ in Thousands," IMS National Sales Perspectives Audit, February 2006, www.imshealth.com, accessed April 7, 2007.
20. Linda Raber, "Tide Honored as Historic Landmark," *Chemical and Engineering News*, vol. 84, no. 47, November 20, 2006, 92.
21. IMS Health, "Leading Products by Global Pharmaceutical Sales, 2006,"

accessed May 1, 2007; www.hoovers.com/levi-strauss—ID_40278—/free-co-factsheet.xhtml, accessed May 8, 2007.

22. Brian Taylor Slingsby, "The Prozac Boom and Its Placebogenic Counterpart—a Culturally Fashioned Phenomenon," Medical Science Monitor, vol. 8, no. 5, 2002, 389–93.
23. Rebecca Segall, "Bye Wonderland," *Psychology Today*, July 1, 2000.
24. Pamela Berard. "Advertising Campaigns Bring Mental Illness to the Forefront," *New England Psychologist*, vol. 15, no. 4, May 2007.
25. O. F. Wahl, "News Media Portrayal of Mental Illness: Implications for Public Policy," *American Behavioral Scientist*, vol. 46, 2003, 1594–1600.
26. D. L. Diefenbach, "The Portrayal of Mental Illness on Prime-Time Television," *Journal of Community Psychology*, vol. 25, 1997, 289–302.
27. Russell McCulley, "Is New Orleans Having a Mental Health Breakdown?" *Time*, August 1, 2006.
28. CNN.com, "Study: Thousands of Veterans Return with Mental Illness," March 13, 2007.
29. Susanna Fox, "Online Health Search 2006," Pew Internet and American Life Project, October 29, 2006, www.pewinternet.org.
30. eMarketer, "Big Pharma Boosts Ad Spending," October 23, 2006, www.emarketer.com, accessed August 15, 2007.
31. Daniel Jacobs, "Depression Is Top Researched Condition Online," *International Business Times*, December 6, 2006, www.ibtimes.com/articles/20061206/depression_searchonline.htm, accessed October 1, 2007.
32. Daniel Goleman, "Flame First, Think Later: New Clues to E-Mail Misbehavior," *The New York Times*, February 20, 2007.
33. Cara Buckley, "Why Our Hero Leapt onto the Tracks and We Might Not," January 7, 2007.
34. Sandra Blakeslee, "Cells That Read Minds," *The New York Times*, January 10, 2006.
35. Science Times, *The New York Times*. All articles cited are from the March 16, 2004, edition of Science Times.
36. Alex Beam, "The Mad Poets Society," *The Atlantic Monthly*, July/August 2001.
37. Katherine A. Kaplan, "College Faces Mental Health Crisis," *Harvard Crimson*, January 12, 2004.

38. Richard Kadison, "Getting an Edge—Use of Stimulants and Antidepressants in College," *New England Journal of Medicine*, vol. 353, no. 11, September 15, 2005, 1089–91.
39. "Uncovering the Real Abe Lincoln," *Time*, July 4, 2005.
40. Todd Leopold, "Putting 'The Sopranos' on the Couch," CNN.com Entertainment, August 28, 2002.
41. "Too Much Money, Too Much Media Say Voters," Pew Research Center for People and the Press, report released September 15, 1999.
42. S. Klineberg, "Public Perceptions of Mental Illness. A Report to the Mental Health Association of Greater Houston," Rice University, 2004.
43. Mental Health America, "10-Year Retrospective Study Shows Progress in American Attitudes about Depression and Other Mental Health Issues," June 6, 2007, www.nmha.org, accessed June 20, 2007.
44. The WHO World Mental Health Survey Consortium, "Prevalence, Severity and Unmet Need for Treatment of Mental Disorders in the World Health Organization World Mental Health Surveys," *Journal of the American Medical Association*, vol. 291, no. 21, June 2, 2004, 2581–90.
45. Benedict Carey, "Most Will Be Mentally Ill at Some Point, Study Says," *The New York Times*, June 7, 2005.
46. Rick Weiss, "Study: U.S. Leads in Mental Illness, Lags in Treatment," *The Washington Post*, June 7, 2005.
47. Matthew Herper, "Big Pharma's Drought," *Forbes*, October 26, 2005.
48. "Leading Therapy Classes by Global Pharmaceutical Sales, 2006"; "Top 10 Therapeutic Classes by U.S. Sales, 2006," www.imshealth.com, accessed August 23, 2007.
49. R. M. Scheffler, S. P. Hinshaw, S. Modrek, and P. Levine, "The Global Market for ADHD Medication," *Health Affairs*, vol. 26, no. 2, March/April 2007: 450–57.
50. Peter Kramer, *Listening to Prozac* (New York: Viking, 1993), p. 274.

CHAPTER TWO: THE COMMERCE OF MOOD

1. David Healy, *The Creation of Psychopharmacology* (Cambridge, MA: Harvard University Press, 2002), p. 2.

2. Marcia Angell, "Excess in the Pharmaceutical Industry," *Canadian Medical Association Journal* vol. 171, no. 12 (December 7, 2004).
3. James Surowiecki, "The Pipeline Problem," *The New Yorker*, February 16 and 23, 2004; "Pharmaceutical Profits Make Us Sick," *The Guardian* (UK), May 8, 2002.
4. "Pharmaceutical Industry Ranks as Most Profitable Industry—Again," A Public Citizen Report, April 18, 2002.
5. Families USA, "Off the Charts: Pay, Profits, and Spending by Drug Companies," July 2001, www.familiesusa.org, accessed September 10, 2007.
6. Families USA, "The Choice: Health Care for People or Drug Industry Profits," September 2005.
7. Fortune 500, 2007.
8. Raghunath Tantry, "Expanding Indication Segments Boost CNS Therapeuetics Markets," Frost & Sullivan, May 15, 2003, http://frost.com, accessed August 23, 2007.
9. Carl Elliott, "Medicate Your Dissent," *Speakeasy*, May/June 2003.
10. Andrew Humphreys and Rebecca Mayer, "World's Best-Selling Medicines," *Med Ad News*, June 7, 2005.
11. IMS Health, "Leading Therapy Classes by Global Pharmaceutical Sales, 2006," www.imshealth.com.
12. Alex Berenson, "Drug Files Show Maker Promoted Unapproved Use," *The New York Times*, December 18, 2006; IMS Health, Leading Products by Global Pharmaceutical Sales 2005.
13. Angela K. Brown, "Questions Raised About Drug Yates Was Taking," *Houston Chronicle*, July 9, 2006.
14. NDC Health, "Top 200 Drugs for 2004 by U.S. Sales," NDC Phast, March 2005, www.drugs.com/top200.html, accessed August 27, 2006.
15. CBS News HealthWatch, "Mother's Little Helper Turns 40," July 16, 2003.
16. Patricia Sullivan, "Creator of Valium Dies at 97," *The Washington Post*, September 30, 2005.
17. Ibid.
18. Joshua Kendall, "Talking Back to Prozac," *The Boston Globe*, February 1, 2004.

19. R. S. Bobrow, "Benzodiazepines Revisited," *Family Practice*, vol. 20, 2003, 347–49.
20. Sullivan, *The Washington Post*.
21. Drug Topics. Top 200 Generic Drugs by Units in 2006. March 5, 2007. www.drugtopics.com/drugtopics/issue/issueDetail.jsp?id=11446, accessed October 5, 2007.
22. Richard Gordon, personal correspondence, August 29, 2006.
23. Harvey Mansfield, "Response to Francis Fukuyama's Second Thoughts: The Last Man in a Bottle," *The National Interest*, Summer 1999.
24. "Pharmaceutical Industry Ranks as Most Profitable Industry—Again."
25. Robert Langreth and Matthew Herper, "Pill Pushers: How the Drug Industry Abandoned Science for Salesmanship," *Forbes*, May 8, 2006.
26. Marcia Angell, "The Truth About the Drug Companies," *The New York Review of Books*, vol. 51, no. 12, July 15, 2004.
27. Marcia Angell, "Excess in the Pharmaceutical Industry," *Canadian Medical Association Journal*, vol. 171, no. 12, December 7, 2004, 1451–53, www.cmaj.ca/cgi/content/full/171/12/1451, accessed August 27, 2007.
28. Jim Drinkard, "Drugmakers Go Furthest to Sway Congress," *USA Today*, April 25, 2005.
29. Milt Freudenheim, "Showdown Looms in Congress over Drug Advertising on TV," *The New York Times*, January 22, 2007.
30. Angell, "The Truth About the Drug Companies."
31. Marc Kaufman, "FDA's Reliance on Unconfirmed Chiefs Is Faulted," *The Washington Post*, December 19, 2004.
32. Statement of Sidney M. Wolfe, director, Public Citizen's Health Research Group, "The 100th Anniversary of the FDA: The Sleeping Watchdog Whose Master Is Increasingly the Regulated Industries," June 27, 2006, www.citizen.org/pressroom/release.cFm?ID-2228, accessed August 27, 2007.
33. The Henry J. Kaiser Family Foundation, Daily Health Policy Reports, Capitol Hill Watch, "Lawmakers Have Not Commented on FDA User Fee Proposal," March 29, 2007, www.kaisernetwork.org.
34. Bill Vaughan, personal correspondence, May 10, 2007.
35. Kaiser Family Foundation, Daily Health Policy Reports, "Lawmakers Have Not Commented," March 29, 2007.

36. Bloomberg.
37. David Evans, Michael Smith, and Liz Willen, "Big Pharma's Shameful Secret," Bloomberg Markets, December 2005.
38. Kaufman, "FDA's Reliance on Unconfirmed Chiefs Is Faulted."
39. CBS News Healthwatch, "Pfizer to Halt Celebrex Ads," December 20, 2004, www.cbsnews.com.
40. Freudenheim, "Showdown Looms in Congress over Drug Advertising on TV."
41. Julie Schmit, "FDA Races to Keep Up with Drug Ads That Go Too Far," *USA Today*, May 30, 2005.
42. "Drug Industry, FDA User-Fee Deal Fails to Fix Drug Safety Crisis: New Laws and Real Funds Are Needed," January 11, 2007, www.consumers union.org.
43. Schmit, *USA Today*.
44. *Frontline*, interview with Sidney Wolfe, "Dangerous Prescription," November 4, 2002, www.pbs.org.
45. Shankar Vedantam, "Antidepressant Makers Withhold Data on Children," *The Washington Post*, January 29, 2004.
46. David Healy, "Evidence Biased Psychiatry?" *Psychiatric Bulletin* 25 (2001): 290–91.
47. Gerard Sanacora MD, personal correspondence, August 20, 2007.
48. Ibid.
49. Jim Rosack, "FDA Panel Rejects New Rule for Psychiatric Drug Testing," *Psychiatric News*, vol. 40, no. 22, November 18, 2005, p. 1.
50. Indrajit Basu, "India's Clinical Trials and Tribulations," *Asia Times*, July 23, 2004.
51. S. G. Damle, "Clinical Trials Beyond the Darker Side," *Journal of Indian Society of Pedodontics and Preventive Dentistry* 24, issue 1 (2006): 6.
52. Basu, "India's Clinical Trials," July 23, 2004.
53. Center for Science in the Public Interest, Press Release, "FDA Fails to Protect Americans from Dangerous Drugs and Unsafe Foods," June 27, 2006, http://cspinet.org/new/200606271.html, accessed July 11, 2007.
54. Angell, "Excess in the Pharmaceutical Industry."

55. Jerome P. Kassirer, "How Drug Lobbyists Influence Doctors," *The Boston Globe*, February 13, 2006.
56. Center for Policy Alternatives, "Prescription Drug Marketing," http://www.stateaction.org/issues/issue.cfm/issue/PrescriptionDrugMarketing.xml, accessed August 26, 2007.
57. Langreth and Herper, "Pill Pushers."
58. Center for Policy Alternatives, "Prescription Drug Marketing," 2007.
59. Ibid.
60. Angell, "Excess in the Pharmaceutical Industry."
61. E. Fuller Torrey, "The Going Rate on Shrinks: Big Pharma and the Buying of Psychiatry," *The American Prospect*, July 15, 2002.
62. Stephanie Saul, "Gimme an Rx! Cheerleaders Pep Up Drug Sales," *The New York Times*, November 28, 2005.
63. Carl Elliott, "The Drug Pushers," *The Atlantic Monthly*, April 31, 2006.
64. Saul, "Gimme an Rx! Cheerleaders Pep Up Drug Sales."
65. Langreth and Herper, "Pill Pushers"
66. Angell, "The Truth About the Drug Companies."
67. Berenson, "Drug Files Show Maker Promoted Unapproved Use."
68. Alex Berenson, "Lilly Settles with 18,000 over Zyprexa," *The New York Times*, January 5, 2007.
69. Ibid.
70. Berenson, "Drug Files Show Maker Promoted Unapproved Use."
71. Alex Berenson, "Lilly Adds Strong Warning Label to Zyprexa, a Schizophrenia Drug," *The New York Times*, October 6, 2007.
72. Berenson, "Drug Files Show Maker Promoted Unapproved Use."
73. Department of Justice, "Warner-Lambert to Pay $430 Million to Resolve Criminal and Civil Health Care Liability Relating to Off-Label Promotion," May 13, 2004, www.usdoj.gov/opa/pr/2004/May/04_civ_322.htm, accessed October 10, 2007.
74. 101 Facts About Clinical Research. The Center for Information and Study on Clinical Research Participation, July 2005, www.ciscrp. org/information/documents/101FactsAboutClinicalResearch.pdf, accessed August 8, 2007.
75. R. H. Perlis, C. S. Perlis, Y. Wu, C. Hwang, M. Joseph, A. A. Nierenberg, "Industry Sponsorship and Financial Conflict of Interest in the Reporting

of Clinical Trials in Psychiatry," *American Journal of Psychiatry*, vol. 162, October 2005, pp. 1957–60.

76. Langreth and Herper, "Pill Pushers."
77. David Healy, "The Dilemmas Posed by New and Fashionable Treatments," *Advances in Psychiatric Treatment*, vol. 7, 2001, 322–27.
78. Scott Masters, M.D., personal correspondence, June 12, 2007.
79. Daniel Carlat, "Generic Smear Campaign," *New York Times*, May 9, 2006.
80. Adriane Fugh Berman, "Not in My Name; How I Was Asked to 'Author' a Ghostwritten Research Paper," *The Guardian* (UK), April 21, 2005.
81. Ibid.
82. Carl Elliott, "Pharma Goes to the Laundry: Public Relations and the Business of Medical Education," The Hastings Center Report, November 11, 2004.
83. Erica Johnson, CBC Marketplace, "Inside the Business of Medical Ghostwriting," broadcast March 25, 2003, www.cbc.ca/consumers/market/files/health/ghostwriting/, accessed October 21, 2007.
84. Carl Elliott, "Pharma Goes to the Laundry."
85. D. Healy and D. Cattell, "Interface Between Authorship, Industry and Science in the Domain of Therapeutics," *British Journal of Psychiatry* 183, 2003, pp. 22–27; Elliott, "Pharma Goes to the Laundry."
86. Marcia Angell, "Editorial: Is Academic Medicine for Sale?" *New England Journal of Medicine*, vol. 342, no. 20, 2000, 1516–18.
87. Gardiner Harris, "Psychiatrists Top List in Drug Maker Gifts," *The New York Times*, June 26, 2007.
88. Benedict Carey, "Study Finds a Link of Drug Makers to Psychiatrists," *The New York Times*, April 20, 2006.
89. N. K. Choudhry, H. T. Stelfox, and A. S. Detsky, "Relationships Between Authors of Clinical Practice Guidelines and the Pharmaceutical Industry," *Journal of the American Medical Association*, vol. 287, no. 5, 2002, 612–17.
90. Carl Elliott, "Pharma Buys a Conscience," *The American Prospect*, vol. 12, no.17, September 24, 2005–October 8, 2001, 16–20.
91. Research America/Harris Interactive "101 Facts About Clinical Research," www.ciscrip.org/information/documents/101FactsaboutClinicalResearch.pdf, accessed August 15, 2007.

92. Alex Berenson, "Big Drug Makers See Sales Decline with Their Image," *The New York Times*, November 14, 2005.
93. Phyllis Maguire, "How Direct-to-Consumer Advertising Is Putting the Squeeze on Physicians," *ACP-ASIM Observer* (American College of Physicians–American Society of Internal Medicine), March 1999.
94. B. Mintzes, M. L. Barer, R. L. Kravitz, and K. Bassett, "How Does Direct-to-Consumer Advertising (DTCA) Affect Prescribing? A Survey in Primary Care Environments With and Without Legal DTCA," *Canadian Medical Association Journal*, vol. 169, no. 5, September 2003, 405–12.
95. eMarketer, "Big Pharma Boosts Ad Spending," October 23, 2006, www.emarketer.com.
96. R. L. Kravitz, R. M. Epstein, M. D. Feldman, C. E. Franz, et al., "Influence of Patients' Requests for Direct-to-Consumer Advertised Antidepressants," *JAMA*, vol. 293, 2005, 1995–2002.
97. Lisa Richwine, "Prescription Drug Giveaways Draw Complaints," *Boston Globe*, August 13, 2006.
98. Consumer Reports Best Buy Drugs, Update, "New Drug Ads You Should Be Skeptical of—or Ignore," June 2007.
99. Bernard I. Koerner, "Disorders Made to Order," *Mother Jones*, July/August 2002.
100. Christopher Lane, "Shy on Drugs," *The New York Times*, September 21, 2007; "Pharmaceutical Profits Make Us Sick," *The Guardian*, May 2, 2002.
101. IMS Health, "Leading Products by Global Pharmaceutical Sales, 2001," www.imshealth.com.
102. Jim Rosack, "Drug Makers Find Sept. 11 a Marketing Opportunity," *Psychiatric News*, vol. 37, no. 5, March 1, 2002.
103. C. DiMaggio, S. Galea, and P. Madrid, letter: "SSRI Prescription Rates After a Terrorist Attack," *Psychiatric Services*, vol. 57, November 2006, 1656–57.
104. Vanessa O'Connell and Rachel Zimmerman, "Drugmakers Plug Their Pills as the Cure for Americans' Struggle with Grief, Fear," *The Wall Street Journal*, January 14, 2002, as republished by www.drugawareness.org/Archives, accessed October 3, 2007.

105. http://squarefootagefilms.com/smith/commercials.html, accessed October 23, 2007.
106. Kate Arthur, Television: Broadcast, "Little Blob, Don't Be Sad (or Anxious or Phobic)," *The New York Times*, January 2, 2005.
107. Workshop Speakers' Profiles. 2004 Ottawa International Animation Festival. www.awn.com/ottawa/OIAF04/prog-workshop_speakers.html, accessed November 10, 2007.
108. *CNN Paula Zahn Now*, "Who Is Really in Charge of America's Health," aired August 5, 2004, http://transcripts.cnn.com/TRANSCRIPTS/0408/05/pznOD.html, accessed October 23, 2007.
109. Michael Montagne, "Patient Drug Information from Mass Media Sources," *Psychiatric Times*, vol. 19, no 5. May 1, 2002.
110. Robert Ehrlich, DTC Perspectives, personal correspondence, April 9, 2007.
111. John Mack, "Spend, Spend, Spend Before the End, End, End," March 28, 2007, Pharmamarketing Blog, www.pharmamkting.blogspot.com, accessed April 13, 2007.
112. Healy, *Let Them Eat Prozac*, p. 33.
113. Susan Ipaktchian, "The Name Game," *The Patriot Ledger*, June 7, 2005.
114. Donald C. McNeil Jr., "The Science of Naming Drugs (Sorry, 'Z' Is Already Taken)," *New York Times*, December 27, 2003.
115. Ipaktchian, "The Name Game."
116. McNeil, "The Science of Naming Drugs."
117. www.frankdelano.biz/about.html, accessed August 27, 2007.
118. Healy, *Let Them Eat Prozac*, p. 38.
119. Ibid., p. 35–36.
120. Ibid., p. 36.
121. R. Y. Ackerman and J. W. Williams, "Rational Treatment Choices for Non-Major Depressions in Primary Care: An Evidence-based Review," *Journal of General Internal Medicine*, vol. 17, no. 4, 2002, 293–201.
122. Scott Masters, M.D., personal correspondence, June 12, 2007.
123. E. Lewis, S. C. Marcus, M. Olfson, B. G. Druss, H. A. Pincus, "Datapoints: Patients' Early Discontinuation of Antidepressant Prescriptions," *Psychiatric Services*, vol. 55, May 2004, 494.

124. J. M. Pomerantz, "Antidepressants Used as Placebos: Is That Good Practice?" *Drug Benefit Trends*, vol. 15, no. 8, 2003, 32–33.
125. T. Kendrick, editorial: "Prescribing Antidepressants in General Practice," *British Medical Journal*, vol. 313, October 5, 1996, 829–30.
126. Arif Khan and Shirif Khan, "Are Placebo Controls Ethical in Antidepressant Trials?" *Psychiatric Times*, vol. xviii, issue 4, April 2000.
127. Treatment of Depression: Newer Pharmacotherapies, Sumary, Evidence Report/Technology Assessment: Number 7, March 1999, Agency for Health Care Policy and Research, Rockville, MD, http://www.ahrq.gov/clinic/epcsums/deprsumm.htm, accessed January 5, 2005.
128. Oliver Wright, "Crackdown on Antidepressants Given Out 'Like Sweets,' " *The Times* (UK), October 20, 2003.
129. Apoorva Mandavilli, "Mood Swings," *Nature Medicine*, September 8, 2004.
130. C. Sherman, "Long-term Side Effects Surface with SSRIs," *Clinical Psychiatry News*, vol. 26, no. 5, 1998, 1.
131. K. D. Wagner, P. Ambroisine, M. Rynn, and C. Wowhlberg, "Efficacy of Sertraline in the Treatment of Children and Adolescents with Major Depressive Disorder," *JAMA*, 290, August 27, 2003, 1033–41.
132. Sherman, "Long-term Side Effects," 1998.
133. David Healy, "SSRIs & Withdrawal/Dependence," briefing paper, June 20, 2003, www.socialaudit.org.uk/58092-DH.htm, accessed August 23, 2007.
134. Erik Hoencamp, A. Stevens, and J. Haffmans, Letters: "Patients' Attitudes Toward Antidepressants," *Psychiatric Services*, vol. 53, September 2002, 1180–81.
135. C. H. Warner, W. Bobo, C. Warner, S. Reid, and J. Rachal, "Antidepressant Discontinuation Syndrome," *American Family Physician*, vol. 5, 2006, 449–57.
136. Mary Duenwald, "How to Stop Depression Medications: Very Slowly," *The New York Times*, May 25, 2004.
137. C. H. Warner, et al., "Antidepressant Discontinuation Syndrome."
138. A. Preda, R. W. MacLean, C. M. Mazure, and M. B. Bowers, "Antidepressant-Associated Mania and Psychosis Resulting in Psychiatric Admissions," *Journal of Clinical Psychiatry*, vol. 62, no. 1, 2001, 30–33.

139. R. Levinson-Castiel, P. Merlob, N. Linder, et al., "Neonatal Abstinence Syndrome After In-utero Exposure to Selective Serotonin Reuptake Inhibitors in Term Infants," *Archives of Pediatrics and Adolescent Medicine*, vol. 160, 2006, 173–76.
140. Robert Epstein, "Is Everybody Happy? Interview with Peter Kramer," *Psychology Today*, November-December 2001.
141. Harriet Brown, "A Brain in the Head, and One in the Gut," *The New York Times*, August 25, 2005
142. Elliott, "Medicate Your Dissent."
143. Chris Noon, "Faces in the News: Pfizer CEO Takes Home 72% Pay Hike," *Forbes*, March 10, 2005.
144. Moira Herbst, "*The Golden Parachute* Club of 2006," *BusinessWeek*, December 22, 2006.
145. Bill Alpert, "Pill Power," *SmartMoney*, December 1, 2003. www.smartmoney.com/barrows/index.cfm?story=20031201, accessed October 10, 2007.

CHAPTER THREE: THE TRIUMPH OF BIOLOGICAL PSYCHIATRY

1. David Healy, *The Creation of Psychopharmacology* (Cambridge, MA: Harvard University Press, 2002), p. 2.
2. The formulation of the distinct entities of Community and Corporate Psychiatry is David Healy's, from Ibid.
3. Edward Shorter, *A History of Psychiatry from the Era of the Asylum to the Age of Prozac* (New York: John Wiley & Sons, 1997), 34 "Deinstitutionalization: A Psychiatric 'Titanic,' " PBS *Frontline*, www.pbs.org/wgbh/pages/frontline/shows/asylums/special/excerpt.html, accessed August 27, 2007.
4. Jonathan Michel Metzl, *Prozac on the Couch: Prescribing Gender in the Era of Wonder Drugs* (Durham, NC: Duke University Press, 2003), p. 195.
5. Daniel Defoe, "An Essay Upon Projects" (1699), in R. Hunter and I. Macalpine, *Three Hundred Years of Psychiatry* (London: Oxford University Press, 1963).
6. Robert Whitacker, *Mad in America: Bad Science, Bad Medicine and the*

Enduring Mistreatment of the Mentally Ill (New York: Perseus Publishing, 2003), p. 59.

7. Ibid., p. 60.
8. Ibid., p. 62.
9. Ibid., pp. 80–82.
10. Ibid., p. 82.
11. Alex Beam, *Gracefully Insane* (New York: Public Affairs, 2001), pp. 118, 154.
12. Edward Shorter, *A History of Psychiatry: From the Era of the Asylum to the Age of Prozac* (New York: John Wiley & Sons, 1997), p. 211.
13. Whitaker, *Mad in America*, pp. 108, 110–114.
14. Ibid., p. 134.
15. Ibid., p. 124.
16. Leon Eisenberg, editorial: "Is Psychiatry More Mindful or Brainier Than It Was a Decade Ago?" *The British Journal of Psychiatry*, vol. 176: 1–5, 2000.
17. Healy, *The Creation of Psychopharmacology*, p. 140.
18. Shorter, *A History of Psychiatry*, p. 289.
19. Amy Harmon, "That Wild Streak? Maybe It Runs in the Family," *The New York Times*, June 15, 2006.
20. Caroline Hadley, interview with Steven Rose, "The Gene and Its Place," European Molecular Biology Organization (EMBO) Reports, vol. 5, no. 3, 2004, 226–29, www.nature.com/embor/journal/v5/n3, accessed August 1, 2007.
21. David Healy, *The Antidepressant Era* (Cambridge, MA: Harvard University Press, 1997), p. 89.
22. B. Thornley and C. Adams, "Content and Quality of 2000 Controlled Trials in Schizophrenia Over 50 Years," *British Medical Journal*, vol. 317, 1998, 1181–84.
23. Gareth Cook, "Surveyed Scientists Admit Misconduct; One Third Cite Research Tactics," *The Boston Globe*, June 9, 2005.
24. Healy, *The Creation of Psychopharmacology*, ch. 7; David Healy, personal correspondence, March 8, 2007.
25. Ibid., p. 198.

26. Ibid., p. 143.
27. Ibid., p. 175–77.
28. Tom Wolfe, Lecture for the Benefit of the Southampton Public Library, Southampton, New York, Summer 1993.
29. R. Mize, B. R. Talamo, R. I. Schoenfeld, et al., "Neuroscience Training at the Turn of the Century: A Summary Report of the Third Annual ANDP Survey," *Nature Neuroscience*, vol. 3, 2000, 433–35.
30. Eisenberg, "Is Psychiatry More Mindful?"
31. FY 2005 Annual Progress Report: Advancing Scientific Excellence, Society for Neuroscience, *Neuroscience Quarterly*, http://www.sfn.org. (Marlene Poole, director of Membership and Chapters, Society for Neuroscience, personal correspondence, August 30, 2006.)
32. SfN Membership Growth, 1991–2005, Society for Neuroscience/About Membership, http://www.sfn.org.
33. T. M. Luhrmann, *Of Two Minds: An Anthropologist Looks at American Psychiatry* (New York: Vintage, 2000), p. 237.
34. American Psychiatric Association Statement of Diagnosis and Treatment of Mental Disorders, September 25, 2003.
35. Philip Rieff, *Freud: The Mind of a Moralist* (Chicago and London: University of Chicago Press, 1979), p. xi.
36. George Scialabba, "Final Analysis; Book Review of *Secrets of the Soul: A Social and Cultural History of Psychoanalysis*," *The Boston Globe*, July 18, 2004.
37. Shorter, *A History of Psychiatry*, p. 181.
38. Claudia Dreifus, "A Rebel Psychiatrist Calls Out to His Profession," *The New York Times*, August 27, 2002.
39. Healy, *The Creation of Psychopharmacology*, p. 28.
40. Nathan G. Hale Jr., *The Rise and Crisis of Psychoanalysis in the United States* (New York: Oxford University Press, 1995), p. 188.
41. Hale, *The Rise and Crisis*, p. 188.
42. Ibid., p. 188.
43. John C. Burham, *Paths into American Culture* (Philadelphia: Temple University Press, 1988), pp. 100–101.
44. "Are You Always Worrying?" *Time*, October 25, 1948.

45. Hale, *The Rise and Crisis*, pp. 201–2.
46. David Healy, "Psychopharmacology and the Government of the Self," Academy for the Study of the Psychoanalytic Arts, www.academyanalyticarts.org/healy.htm, accessed July 1, 2007.
47. Ibid.
48. Burnham, *Paths into American Culture*, p. 101.
49. Burnham, *Paths into American Culture*, p. 102.
50. Ibid.
51. Hale, *The Rise and Crisis*, p. 289.
52. Ibid.
53. Lawrence J. Friedman, *Menninger* (New York: Alfred A. Knopf, 1990), p. 26; Hale, *The Rise and Crisis*, p. 289.
54. Luhrmann, *Of Two Minds*, p. 214.
55. Ibid.
56. Healy, *The Creation of Psychopharmacology*, p. 143.
57. Shorter, *A History of Psychiatry*, p. 313.
58. Michael Gazzaniga, *The Mind's Past* (Berkeley: University of California Press, 1998), p. 2.
59. Sigmund Freud, *Beyond the Pleasure Principle* (New York: Norton, 1990), originally published in 1920.
60. Healy, *The Creation of Psychopharmacology*, pp. 4, 255, 341; Shorter, *A History of Psychiatry*, p. 255.
61. People and Discoveries: Drugs for Treating Schizophrenia Identified, 1952, Public Broadcasting Service, www.pbs.org/wgbh/aso/databank/entries/dh52dsr.html, accessed October 1, 2007.
62. Shorter, p. 254.
63. Ibid.
64. Healy, *The Creation of Psychopharmacology*, p. 241.
65. Joseph T. Coyle and Daniel C. Javitt, "Decoding Schizophrenia: A Fuller Understanding of Signaling in the Brain of People with this Disorder Offers Improved Treatment," *Scientific American*, January 2004.
66. Healy, p. 255.
67. People and Discoveries.
68. Shorter, *A History of Psychiatry*, p. 280.

69. Ibid., p. 308.
70. Nancy C. Andreasen, M.D., Ph.D., "O Brave New World! Exploring the Mind and Brain in Health and Disease," a presidential lecture, University of Iowa, 1993. http://sdrc.lib.uiowa/preslectures/andreasen93/index/html, accessed October 10, 2007.
71. Mark S. George, "Advances in Brain Imaging: An Overview of What the Primary Psychiatrist Needs to Know," Medical University of South Carolina, www.musc.edu/fnrd/primer_overview.htm, accessed September 5, 2007.
72. Stephen Pinker, "Will the Mind Figure Out How the Brain Works, *Time*, October 26, 2004.
73. Sharon Begley, "While Brain Imaging Offers New Knowledge, It Can Be an Illusion," *The Wall Street Journal*, March 18, 2005.
74. The President's Council on Bioethics (PCBE): Transcripts (June 25, 2004): Neuroscience, Brain, and Behavior IV: Brain Imaging (Case Study).
75. Carey, "Can Brain Scans See Depression?"
76. Amy Harmon, "Neurodiversity Forever: The Disability Movement Turns to Brains," *New York Times*, May 9, 2004.
77. John Tierney, "Using M.R.I's to See Politics on the Brain," *The New York Times*, April 20, 2004.
78. Gary Stix, "Ultimate Self-Improvement," *Scientific American*, September 2003, pp. 44–46.
79. Elio Frattaroli, *Healing the Soul in the Age of the Brain* (New York: Viking, 2001), p. 7.
80. Darby Saxbe, "Placebo Power: A Mystery Grows," *Psychology Today*, September-October 2004.
81. Mark Sappenfield, "India Poised for Pharmaceutical Boom," *The Christian Science Monitor*; January 2, 2007
82. Marialba Martinez, "Caribbean Business: Local Manufacturing of Pfizer/Pharmacia Products Yields $25.8 Billion in 2002 Sales: Thirteen of 26 Key Products Manufactured in Puerto Rico," *Puerto Rico Herald*, March 13, 2003.
83. David Healy, *The Creation of Psychopharmacology*, (Cambridge, MA: Harvard University Press, 2002), p. 173.

84. "More Than a Million Kids on Psychotropic Medication," *Reno Gazette Journal,* March 4, 2004.
85. Gogo Lidz, "My Adventures in Psychopharmacology," *New York* magazine, January 8, 2007.
86. Benedict Carey, "Use of Antipsychotics by the Young Rose Fivefold," *The New York Times,* June 6, 2006.
87. Gardiner Harris, "Sleeping Pill Use by Youths Soars, Study Says," *The New York Times,* October 19, 2005.
88. Ibid.
89. Michael D. Lemonick, "In Our Streams: Prozac and Pesticides," *Time,* August 25, 2003.
90. Betsy Mason, "River Fish Accumulate Human Drugs," *Nature News Service,* November 5, 2003, www.nature.com/nsu031103/031103-8.html, accessed August 20, 2007.
91. Marsha Walton, "Frogs, Fish and Pharmaceuticals a Troubling Brew," CNN.com, November 14, 2003, http://edition.cnn.com/2003/TECH/science/11/14/coolsc/frogs/fish/index.html, accessed August 26, 2007.
92. Tom Arrandale, "Prozac in the Water," *Governing Magazine,* vol. 19, no. 12, September 2006, 56–58.
93. Percy Walker, *The Thanatos Syndrome* (New York: Farrar Straus and Giroux, 1987).
94. NIH News, "Research Identifies Proteins Crucial to Construction of Brain's Information Superhighway," National Institutes of Health, press release, February 10, 2005.
95. Eric Kandel, "A New Intellectual Framework for Psychiatry," *American Journal of Psychiatry,* vol. 155, no. 44, 1998, 457–69.
96. John Horgan, *The Undiscovered Mind: How the Human Brain Defies Replication, Medication, and Explanation* (New York: The Free Press, 1999), p. 19.
97. J. R. Lacasse and J. Leo, "Serotonin and Depression: A Disconnect Between the Advertisements and the Scientific Literature," PLoS Med 2 (12): e392, doi: 10.1371/journal.pmed.0020392, accessed November 11, 2007.
98. L. Iverson, review of *The Psychopharmacologists, Science,* vol. 275, 1997, pp. 1438–39.
99. R. S. Duman, S. Nakagawa, and J. Malberg, "Regulation of Adult Neuro-

genesis by Antidepressant Treatment," *Neuropsychopharmacology*, vol. 2, 2001, 836–44.

100. "Link Between Serotonin and Suicide Found with New Brain Imaging Methods," Centre for Addiction and Mental Health, University of Toronto, press release, January 1, 2003.
101. Shorter, *A History of Psychiatry*, p. 267.
102. Abram Katz, "Delving in Depression," *New Haven Register*, December 31, 2006.

CHAPTER FOUR: AMERICAN MISERY

1. M. J. Larson, K. Miller, and K. J. Fleming, "Datapoints: Antidepressant Medication Use in Private Insurance Health Plans, 2002," *Psychiatric Services*, vol. 57, no. 175, February 2006.
2. H. Ashton, "Psychotropic Drug Prescribing for Women," *British Journal of Psychiatry*, vol. 158, suppl. 10, 1991, 30–35
3. Shankar Vedantam, "Antidepressant Use by U.S. Adults Soars," *The Washington Post*, December 3, 2004.
4. Denise Grady and Gardiner Harris, "Overprescribing Prompted Warning on Antidepressants," *The New York Times*, March 24, 2004.
5. B. Mintzes, et al., "How Does Direct-to-Consumer Advertising (DTCA) Affect Prescribing? A Survey in Primary Care Environments with and Without Legal DTCA," *Canadian Medical Association Journal*, vol. 169, no. 5, September 2003, 405–12.
6. *DTC Perspectives Magazine* (from Reuters Health), "Drug Ads Spur 20 Percent of Consumers to Call Doc," October 10, 2002, www.dtcperspectives.com/contentasp?id=119, accessed August 20, 2007.
7. Nicholas Bakalar, "Doctors Prescribe More Than They Explain," *The New York Times*, October 3, 2006.
8. H. Jick, J. A. Kaye, and S. S. Jick, "Antidepressants and the Risk of Suicidal Behaviors" *Journal of the American Medical Association*, vol. 292, 2004, 338–43.
9. Linda A. Johnson, "Study: No Therapy for Patients on Antidepressants," *The Washington Post*, August 9, 2006.

10. Bruce Stutz, "Self-Nonmedication," *The New York Times Sunday Magazine*, May 6, 2007.
11. Olfson, et al., "National Trends in the Outpatient Treatment of Depression."
12. M. M. Weissman, H. Verdeli, M. J. Gameroff, S. E. Bledsoe, et al., "National Survey of Psychotherapy Training in Psychiatry, Psychology and Social Work," *Archives of General Psychiatry*, vol. 63, 2006, 925–34.
13. Ashley Pettus, "Psychiatry by Prescription," *Harvard Magazine*, July-August 2006.
14. Coeli Carr, "Mental Health Therapists Face Financial Stress as Fees Stagnate," *The New York Times*, March 26, 2006.
15. W. R. Street, "A Chronology of Noteworthy Events in American Psychology," 1994, Washington, DC: American Psychological Association, Addenda, http://www.cwu.edu/-warren/addenda/html, accessed July 10, 2007.
16. Timothy B. McCall, physician commentator, author of *Examining Your Doctor*, on National Public Radio, May 20, 1998, Biopsychiatry Illuminated, www.adhd-report.com/biopsychiatry.bio_32.html, accessed September 12, 2007.
17. Paul Chodoff, "Psychiatric Diagnosis: A 60-Year Perspective," *Psychiatric News*, vol. 40, no. 11, June 3, 2005, 17.
18. M. J. Larson, K. Miller, and K. J. Fleming, "Treatment with Antidepressant Medications in Private Health Plans, *Administration and Policy in Mental Health and Mental Health Services Research*, vol. 34, no. 2, March 2007, 116–26.
19. H. Chen, J. H. Reeves, J. E. Fincham, W. K. Kennedy, J. H. Dorfman, and B. C. Martin, "Off-Label Use of Antidepressant, Anticonvulsant, and Antipsychotic Medications Among Georgia Medicaid Enrollees in 2001," *Journal of Clinical Psychiatry*, vol. 67, no. 6, June 2006, 972–82.
20. Medical News Today. "UGA Researchers Find High Rates of Off-Label Prescriptions: Antidepressant, Anticonvulsant, and Antipsychotic Drugs," July 28, 2006. www.medicalnewstoday.com/articles/48087.php.
21. Allison Young and Chris Adams, "Prescription for Trouble: Approved Medicine Is Being Used for the Wrong Purpose," *Detroit Free Press*, December 3, 2003.
22. Centers for Disease Control, Mental Health Disorders, National

Hospital Ambulatory Medical Care Survey: 2004 Outpatient Department Summary. Table 11, www.cdc.gov/nchs/fastats/mental.htm, accessed August 20, 2007.

23. Martin Seligman Forum on Depression, interview by Julie McGrossin, *Life Matters*, Radio National (Australia), August 16, 2002, www.abc.net.au/rn/talks/lm/stories/s648530.htm.

24. William Styron, *Darkness Visible: A Memoir of Madness* (New York: Vintage Books, 1990).

25. Kay S. Hymowitz, review of *The Mind Has Mountains: Reflections on Society and Psychiatry*, by Paul R. McHugh, *Commentary*, July-August 2006.

26. Sandra J. Ackerman, "The Neurobiology of Suicide." *Brainwork. The Neuroscience Newsletter*, vol. 7, no. 1, January/February 1997.

27. William James, *The Varieties of Religious Experience: A Study in Human Nature* (New York: Lougman, Green and Co., 1905), p. 159.

28. Centers for Disease Control, "Mental Health Disorders. National Ambulatory Medical Care Survey: 2003," www.cdc.gov/nchs/fastats/mental .htm, accessed August 27, 2007; J. C. Coyne, T. L. Schwenk, and S. Fechner-Bates, "Nondetection of Depression by Primary Care Physicians Reconsidered," *General Hospital Psychiatry*, vol. 17, no. 1, January 1995, 3–12.

29. H. U. Wittehen, R. C. Kessler, and K. Beesdo, "Generalized Anxiety and Depression in Primary Care: Prevalence, Recognition, and Management," *Journal of Clinical Psychiatry*, vol. 63, 2002, suppl. 8: 24, 34.

30. J. H. Riskind, A. T. Beck, R. J. Berchick, "Reliability of DSM-III Diagnoses for Major Depression and Generalized Anxiety Disorder Using the Structured Clinical Interview for DSM-III," *Archives of General Psychiatry* vol. 44, no. 9 (September 1987).

31. Joshua Kendall, "Talking Back to Prozac," *Boston Globe*, February 1, 2004.

32. Benedict Carey, "Many Diagnoses of Depression May Be Misguided, Study Says," *The New York Times*, April 3, 2007.

33. Office of Applied Studies, "Serious Psychological Distress in Past Year," SAMHSA, U.S. Department of Health, www.oassamhsa.gov/2k5state/DCMH.htm, accessed August 23, 2007.

34. Mario Maj, *Psychiatric Diagnosis and Classification* (New York: John Wiley & Sons, 2002), p. 48.

35. Jeffrey Oliver, "The Myth of Thomas Szasz," *The New Atlantis: A Journal of Technology and Society*, Summer 2006, pp. 68–84.
36. Elliott, "Medicate Your Dissent." Elliott, "A World of Our Own Making."
37. Shorter, *A History of Psychiatry*, p. 272.
38. R. Moynihan, I. Heath, and D. Henry, "Selling Sickness: The Pharmaceutical Industry and Disease Mongering," *British Medical Journal*, vol. 324, 2002, pp. 886–91.
39. Eve Bender, "In Many Countries Millions Lack Needed MH Care," *Psychiatric News*, vol. 39, no. 17, September 3, 2004, 22.
40. Edward Shorter, "So Many Left Out: The Seriously Ill Lose Out to the Zoloft Set," *Newsday*, August 10, 2003.
41. Treatment Advocacy Center, briefing paper: "What Percentage of Individuals with Severe Mental Illness Are Untreated and Why?" updated April 2007, www.treatmentadvocacycenter.org/briefingpapers/BP13.htm, acessed May 1, 2007.
42. Donald G. McNeil Jr., "Large Study on Mental Illness Funds Global Prevalence," *The New York Times*, June 2, 2004.
43. Philip S. Wang, Olga Demler, and Ronald C. Kessler, "Adequacy of Treatment for Serious Mental Illness in the United States," *American Journal of Public Health*, vol 92, no. 1, January 2002, 92–98.
44. Ibid.
45. L. A. Teplin, G. M. McClelland, K. M. Abram, and D. A. Weiner, "Crime Victimization in Adults with Severe Mental Illness," *Archives of General Psychiatry*, vol. 62, 2005, pp. 911–21.
46. BBC Online News, "Murder Risk Higher for Mentally Ill," December 21, 2001, http://news.bbc.co.uk/1/hi/health/1721156.stm, accessed December 1, 2006
47. Martha Irvine, "A New View of the Mentally Ill: Study Finds Patients No More Violent than Others," CBS News Healthwatch, 1998, www.cbsnews.com/stories/1998/05/14/health/printable9456.shtml, accessed August 25, 2007.
48. "Schizophrenia Research at the NIMH," NIH Publication No. 99-4500, 1999; updated: August 24, 2000.
49. J. J. Mann, "Neurobiology of Suicidal Behavior," *Nature Reviews: Neuroscience*, vol. 4, October 2003, 819–28.

50. Alix Spiegel, "The Dictionary of Disorder," *The New Yorker,* January 3, 2005.
51. J. Angst, K. R. Merikangas, and M. Preisig, "Subthreshold Syndromes of Depression and Anxiety in the Community," *Journal of Clinical Psychiatry,* vol. 58, suppl. 8, 1997, 6–10.
52. Spiegel, "The Dictionary of Disorder."
53. Robin Marantz Henig, "Sorry, Your Eating Disorder Doesn't Meet Our Criteria," *The New York Times,* November 30, 2004.
54. Ray Moynihan, "Scientists Find New Disease: Motivational Deficiency Disorder," *British Medical Journal,* vol. 332, April 1, 2006, 745.
55. Steve Mirsky, "Up the Lazy Creek," *Scientific American,* June 2006.
56. R. C. Kessler, E. F. Coccaro, M. Fava, et al., "The Prevalence and Correlates of DSM-IV Intermittent Explosive Disorder in the National Comorbidity Survey Replication," *Archives of General Psychiatry,* vol. 63, no. 6, June 2006, pp. 669–78.
57. Bruce Bower, "All the Rage: Survey Extends Reach of Explosive-Anger Disorder," *Science News,* June 10, 2006.
58. Chris Berdik, "Selling the Cure for Shopaholism," *Mother Jones,* May 23, 2000.
59. Ed Diener and Martin E. P. Seligman, "Beyond Money: Toward an Economy of Well-Being," *Psychological Science in the Public Interest,* vol. 5, issue 1, July 2004, p. 1.
60. Martin Seligman Forum on Depression, interview by Julie McGrossin.
61. Putnam, *Bowling Alone,* p. 331.
62. Sharon Waxman, "Study Finds Young Men Attending Fewer Films," *New York Times,* October 8, 2005.
63. Robert J. Samuelson, *The Good Life and Its Discontents: The American Dream in the Age of Enlightenment 1945–1995* (New York: Times Books, Random House, 1995), p. 46.
64. Ibid., p. 39.
65. Ibid., p. 7.
66. Ibid., p. 39.
67. Annual Statistical Supplement, 2005. Medicare: Enrollment, Utilization, and Reimbursement. Table 8.B1—Hospital Insurance and/or Supple-

mentary Medical Insurance: Aged persons enrolled, served, and amount reimbursed, by type of coverage and service, selected years 1967–2002, www.ssa.gov/policy/docs/statcomps/supplement/2005/8b.html, accessed August 4, 2006

68. Darrin M. McMahon, "A Right, From the Start," *The Wall Street Journal*, July 1, 2005.
69. Frederick Jackson Turner, *The Frontier in American History* (New York: Henry Holt and Company, 1920) pp. 2–3.

CHAPTER FIVE: *COGITO, ERGO SUM*

1. "A Pioneer in Psychotherapy Research: Aaron Beck," interview by Sidney Bloch, *Australian and New Zealand Journal of Psychiatry*, vol. 38, nos. 11–12, November 2004, 855–67.
2. In session with Judith S. Beck, PhD: Cognitive Behavioral Therapy, interview by Norman Sussman, *Primary Psychiatry*, vol. 13, no. 4, 2006, 31–34.
3. Aaron T. Beck, home page, University of Pennsylvania Health System, mail.med.upenn.edu/~abeck.research.htm, accessed April 10, 2007.
4. Judith S. Beck, *Cognitive Therapy: Basics and Beyond* (New York: Guilford Press, 1995), 18.
5. Ibid.
6. Erica Goode, "A Pragmatic Man and His No-Nonsense Therapy," *The New York Times*, January 11, 2000.
7. "A Pioneer in Psychotherapy Research: Aaron Beck."
8. "Cognitive Therapy Today," Beck Institute's blog, Judith S. Beck writes in: "Self-Disclosure in Cognitive Therapy," January 8, 2007, www.cttoday.org/?p=146, accessed August 26, 2007.
9. S. J. Rupke, D. Blecke, and M. Renfrow, "Cognitive Therapy for Depression," *American Family Physician*, vol. 73, no. 1, January 1, 2006.
10. R. J. DeRubeis, S. D. Hollon, J. D. Amsterdam, R. C. Shelton, et al., "Cognitive Therapy vs. Medications in the Treatment of Moderate to Severe Depression," *Archives of General Psychiatry*, vol. 62, 2005, 409–16;

R. J. DeRubeis, L. Gelfand, T. Z. Tang, and A. D. Simons, "Medications versus Cognitive Behavior Therapy for Severely Depressed Outpatients: Meta-Analysis of Four Randomized Comparisons," *American Journal of Psychiatry*, vol. 156, 1999, 1007–13.

11. Robert Langreth, "Patient, Fix Thyself," *Forbes*, April 9, 2007, 80–86.
12. S. J. Rupke et al., "Cognitive Therapy for Depression."
13. Jay M. Pomerantz, "Focused Psychotherapy as an Alternative to Long-Term Medication," Drug Benefit Trends, 11(7):2-BH-5-BH, 1999.
14. John Hunsley, "The Cost Effectiveness of Psychological Interventions," *Canadian Psychological Association*, May 2002, www.cpa.ca/documents/cost-effectiveness.pdf, accessed October 10, 2007.
15. D. H. Lam, P. Hayward, E. R. Watkins, K. Wright, et al., "Relapse Prevention in Patients with Bipolar Disorder: Cognitive Therapy Outcome After 2 Years," *American Journal of Psychiatry*, vol. 162, no. 2, 2005, pp. 324–29.
16. University of Pennsylvania, "Cognitive Therapy Works as Well as Antidepressants but with Lasting Effects After Therapy Ends," press release, April 4, 2005.
17. Shankar Vedantam, "Drug Ads Hyping Anxiety Make Some Uneasy," *The Washington Post*, July 16, 2001.
18. National Institutes of Mental Health, "Cognitive Therapy Reduced Repeat Suicide Attempts by 50 Percent," press release, August 2, 2005.
19. K. A. Robb, J. E. Williams, V. Duvivier, and D. J. A. Newham, "Pain Management Program for Chronic Cancer-Treatment-Related Pain. A Preliminary Study," *Journal of Pain*, vol. 7, 2006, 82–90.
20. Francis T. Cullen and Paul Gendreau, "From Nothing Works to What Works: Changing Professional Ideology in the 21st Century," *Prison Journal*, vol. 81, no. 3, 2001, 313–38; Robert Ross and Paul Gendreau, eds., *Effective Correctional Treatment* (Toronto: Butterworths Publishing, 1980).
21. Lori Golden, *Evaluation of the Efficacy of a Cognitive-Behavioral Program for Offenders on Probation: Thinking for a Change* (Dallas: University of Texas Southwestern Medical Center, 2002); citing Steve Aos, et al., "The Comparative Costs and Benefits of Programs to Reduce Crime: A Review of National Research Findings with Implications for Washing-

ton State," Washington State Institute for Public Policy, 1999, doc. no. 99-05-1202.

22. *House Arrest*, episode 24, March 26, 2000.

23. Dr. Lewis Opler, personal correspondence, April 12, 2006.

24. John McKenzie, "Fish Oil Helps Treat Depression. Study: Fish Oil Contains Natural Ingredient That Helps Treat Depression," ABC News, August 19, 2006, http://abcnews.go.com.

25. Stephen Mihm, "Does Eating Salmon Lower the Murder Rate?" *The New York Times*, April 16, 2006.

26. J. A. Blumenthal, M. A. Babyak, K. A. Moore, W. A. Craighead, S. Herman, et al., "Effects of Exercise Training on Older Adults with Major Depression," *Archives of Internal Medicine*, vol. 159, 1999, 2349–56.

27. M. Babyak, J. A. Blumenthal, S. Herman, P. Khatri, et al., "Exercise Treatment for Major Depression: Maintenance of Therapeutic Benefit at 10 Months," *Psychosomatic Medicine*, vol. 62, 2000, 633–38.

28. M. J. Lambert and A. E. Bergin, "The Effectiveness of Psychotherapy," in A. Bergin and S. Garfield, eds., *Handbook of Psychotherapy & Behavior Change*, 4th ed. (New York: John Wiley & Sons, 1994), pp. 141–50.

29. G. E. Hogarty, C. M. Anderson, D. J. Reiss, and S. J. Kornblith, "The Environmental-Personal Indicators in the Course of Schizophrenia (EPICS) Research Group: Family Psychoeducation, Social Skills Training, and Maintenance Chemotherapy in the Aftercare Treatment of Schizophrenia. II: Two-Year Effects of a Controlled Study on Relapse and Adjustment," *Archives of General Psychiatry*, vol. 48, 1991, 340–47.

30. P. Fonagy and M. Target, "Predictors of Outcome in Child Psychoanalysis: A Retrospective Study of 763 Cases at the Anna Freud Centre," *Journal of the American Psychoanalytic Association*, vol. 44, 1996, 27–77; M. Target and P. Fonagy, "Efficacy of Psychoanalysis for Children with Emotional Disorders," *Journal of the American Academy of Child & Adolescent Psychiatry*, vol. 33, 1994, 1134–44.

31. Daniel Goleman, *Social Intelligence: The New Science of Human Relationships* (New York: Bantam Books, 2006), p. 247.

32. Ibid., p. 229.

33. G. Gabbard, S. G. Lazar, J. Hornberger, and D. Spiegel, "The Economic

Impact of Psychotherapy: A Review," *American Journal of Psychiatry*, vol. 154, 1997, 147–55.

34. A. Zients, Presentation to the Mental Health Work Group, White House Task Force for National Health Care Reform, April 23, 1993.
35. M. Linehan, H. E. Armstrong, A. Suarez, and D. Allman, "A Cognitive-Behavioral Treatment of Chronically Parasuicidal Borderline Patients," *Archives of General Psychiatry*, vol. 48, 1991, 1060–64. J. Stevenson, and R. Meares, "An Outcome Study of Psychotherapy for Patients with Borderline Personality Disorder," *American Journal of Psychiatry*, vol. 149, 1992, 358–62.
36. Glen O. Gabbard and Susan G. Lazar, "Efficacy and Cost Effectiveness of Psychotherapy," posted on American Psychiatric Association Web site, www.psych.org/psych_practice/ispe_efficacy.htm, accessed August 27, 2007.
37. M. Sijbrandij, M. Olff, J. B. Reitsma, I. V. Carlier, and B. P. Gersons, "Emotional or Educational Debriefing After Psychological Trauma. Randomised Controlled Trial," *British Journal of Psychiatry*, vol. 189, August 2006, 150–5.
38. Langreth, "Patient, Fix Thyself."
39. Bruce Stutz, "Self-nonmedication," *The New York Times*, May 6, 2007.
40. Alexander Linklater and Robert Harland, "After Freud," *Prospect Magazine* (UK), issue 123, June 2006.
41. Langreth, "Patient, Fix Thyself."
42. M. M. Weissman, H. Verdeli, M. J. Gameroff, S. E. Bledsoe, et al., "National Survey of Psychotherapy Training in Psychiatry, Psychology and Social Work," *Archives of General Psychiatry*, vol. 63, 2006, 925–34.
43. SocietyGuardian.co.uk, September 14, 2005.
44. Richard Layard, "Mental Illness Is Now Our Biggest Social Problem," September 14, 2005, SocietyGuardian.co.uk.
45. Adam Brimelow, "Demand for NHS 'Therapy Network,' " BBC Radio, November 22, 2005.
46. Clive J. Robins. "Zen Principles and Mindfulness Practice in Dialectical Behavioral Therapy," *Cognitive and Behavioral Practice*, vol. 9, 2002, 50–57.

47. Dalai Lama, *Ethics for a New Millennium* (New York: Riverhead Books, 1999).
48. Credit to Katy Butler, *Psychotherapy Networker*, for these examples.
49. "Borderline Personality Disorder: Raising Questions, Finding Answers," National Institute of Mental Health, 2001, www.nimh.nih.gov/publicat/bpd.cfm.
50. M. C. Zanarini, "Childhood Experiences Associated with the Development of Borderline Personality Disorder," *Psychiatric Clinics of North America*, vol. 23, no. 1, 2000, 89–101.
51. Nancy Wick, "A UW Professor's New Therapy Is Being Hailed as a Breakthrough in Treating Self-Destructive Patients Who Live Their Lives on the Borderline," *The University of Washington Alumni Magazine*, December 2005.
52. Marsh M. Linehan, *Cognitive-Behavioral Treatment of Borderline Personality Disorder* (New York: Guilford Press, 1993), p. 145.
53. Transcript of interview with Dr. Marsha Linehan, "Borderline Personality Disorder," The Infinite Mind, National Public Radio, www.brtc.psych.washington.edu/res/Borderline, accessed August 1, 2007.
54. M. M. Linehan, H. Schmidt, L. A. Dimeff, et al., "Dialectical Behavior Therapy for Patients with Borderline Personality Disorder and Drug-dependence," *American Journal of Addictions*, vol. 8, no. 4, 1999, 279–92; M. M. Linehan, D. A. Tutek, H. L. Heard, and H. E. Armstrong, "Interpersonal Outcome of Cognitive Behavioral Treatment for Chronically Suicidal Borderline Patients, *American Journal of Psychiatry*, vol. 151, no. 12, 1994, 1771–76; M. M. Linehan, K. A. Comtois, A. M. Murray, et al., "Two-Year Randomized Controlled Trial and Follow-up of Dialectical Behavior Therapy vs. Therapy by Experts for Suicidal Behaviors and Borderline Personality Disorder," *Archives of General Psychiatry*, vol. 63, 2006, 757–66.
55. Wick, "Dangerous Minds: A UW Professor's New Therapy Is Being Hailed as a Breakthrough."
56. A. T. Beck, "Reflections on My Public Dialog with the Dalai Lama." *Cognitive Therapy Today*, 10(1), 1–4, 2005, http://www.beckinstitute.org/InfoID/465/RedirectPath/Add1/FolderID/238/sessi, accessed October 24, 2007.
57. Langreth, "Patient, Fix Thyself."

CHAPTER SIX: THE HUMAN FACTOR

1. Carlo DiClemente, personal correspondence, December 10, 2006.
2. Carlo C. DiClemente, *Addiction and Change: How Addictions Develop and Addicted People Recover* (New York and London: Guilford Press, 2003), p. 30.
3. C. C. DiClemente and C. W. Scott, "Stages of Change: Interactions with Treatment Compliance and Involvement," in L. S. Onken, J. D. Blaine, and J. J. Boren, eds., *Beyond the Therapeutic Alliance: Keeping the Drug-Dependent Individual in Treatment*, NIDA Research Monograph series, no. 165, Rockville, MD, National Institute on Drug Abuse, 1997, pp. 131–56.
4. Miller, personal correspondence.
5. "Enhancing Motivation for Change in Substance Abuse Treatment," Treatment Improvement Protocol (TIP) Series 35, U.S. Department of Health and Human Services, Public Health Service, Substance Abuse and MentalHealth Services Administration, Center for Substance Abuse Treatment, Publication No. (SMA) 99-3354, 1999, p. 2, William R. Miller, Consensus Panel chair.
6. Ibid.
7. Ibid.
8. W. R. Miller, A. Zweben, and C. C. DiClemente, *Motivational Enhancement Therapy Manual: A Clinical Research Guide for Therapists Treating Individuals with Alcohol Abuse and Dependence*, Project MATCH Monograph series, vol. 2, NIH Pub. No. 94-3723, Rockville, MD: National Institute on Alcohol Abuse and Alcoholism, 1995 c.
9. W. R. Miller and S. Rollnick, *Motivational Interviewing: Preparing People for Change*, 1991, p. 75.
10. William Miller, personal correspondence, June 10, 2007.
11. Ibid.
12. Ibid.
13. Richard M. Ryan and Edward L. Deci, "Self-Determination Theory and the Facilitation of Intrinsic Motivation, Social Development and Well-Being," *American Psychologist*, vol. 55, no. 1, January 2000, 68–78.
14. H. Arkowitz and H. A. Westra, "Integrating Motivational Interview-

ing and Cognitive Behavioral Therapy in the Treatment of Depression and Anxiety," *Journal of Cognitive Psychotherapy*, vol. 18, no. 4, 2004, 337–50.

15. Hal Arkowitz, Henry A. Westra, William R. Miller, and Stephen Rollnick, eds., *Motivational Interviewing in the Treatment of Psychological Problems*, (New York: Guilford Press: 2007), in press.

16. Peer Specialist Alliance of America Is Created, www.peersupport.org/LatestNews.htm, accessed October 12, 2007.

17. D. MacKenzie, *The Appleton Temporary Home: A Record of Work* (Boston: T. R. Marvin and Sons, 1875).

18. H. S. Perry, *Psychiatrist of America: The Life of Harry Stack Sullivan* (Cambridge, MA: Harvard University Press, 1982).

19. "Peer Specialist Alliance of America Is Created," http://www.peersupport.org/LatestNews.htm, accessed July 10, 2007; Dr. Larry Davidson, personal correspondence, May 24, 2007.

20. D. Sells, L. Davidson, C. Jewell, M. Rowe, et al., "The Treatment Relationship in Peer-Based and Regular Case Management for Clients with Severe Mental Illness," *Psychiatric Services*, vol. 57, no. 8, August 2006, 1179–84.

21. World Health Organization, World Health Reports 2001, Mental Health: New Understanding, New Hope, www.who.int/whr/2001/en/, accessed November 8, 2007.

22. Patrick A. McGuire, "New Hope for People with Schizophrenia," *Monitor on Psychology*, American Psychological Association, vol. 31, no. 2, February 2000, www.apa.org/monitor/feb00/schizophrenia.html, accessed December 20, 2006.

23. Ibid.

24. Ibid.

25. L. Davidson, D. A. Stayner, S. Lambert, P. Smith, and W. H. Sledge, "Phenomenological and Participatory Research on Schizophrenia: Recovering the Person in Theory and Practice," *Journal of Social Issues*, vol. 53, 1997, 767–84, reprinted in D. L. Tolman and M., Brydon-Miller eds., *From Subjects to Subjectivities: A Handbook of Interpretive and Participatory Methods* (New York: New York University Press, 2001), pp. 163–179;

L. Davidson, D. A. Stayner, C. Nickou, T. H. Stryon, M. Rowe, and M. J. Chinman, "Simply to Be Let In": Inclusion as a Basis for Recovery from Mental Illness," *Psychiatric Rehabilitation Journal*, vol. 24, 2001, 275–88.

26. World Health Organization, *Schizophrenia: An International Follow-up Study* (New York, John Wiley & Sons, 1979); N. Sartorius, A. Jablensky, A. Korten, et al., "Early Manifestations and First-Contact Incidence of Schizophrenia in Different Cultures," *Psychological Medicine*, vol. 16, 1986, 909–28; A. Jablensky, N. Sartorius, G. Ernberg, et al., "Schizophrenia: Manifestations, Incidence and Course in Different Cultures. A World Health Organization Ten-Country Study," *Psychological Medicine*, Monograph Supplement 20, 1992, 1–97.
27. McGuire, "New Hope for People with Schizophrenia."
28. G. E. Vaillant, "Mental Health," *American Journal of Psychiatry*, vol. 160, no. 9, August 2003, 1373–84.
29. E. H. Erikson, "Growth and Crises of the 'Healthy Personality,' in Symposium on the Healthy Personality: Supplement II of the Fourth Conference on Infancy and Childhood," ed. M. J. R. Senn (New York: Josiah Macy Jr. Foundation, 1950), p. 93.
30. J. S. Strauss, "Subjective Experiences of Schizophrenia: Toward a New Dynamic Psychiatry—II," *Schizophrenia Bulletin*, vol. 15, 1989, 182.
31. Dr. Larry Davidson, personal correspondence, May, 24, 2007.
32. Mary Ellen Copeland, "Being the Expert on Yourself," reprinted by permission from HelpHorizons.com, www.helphorizons.com, www.mentalhealthrecovery.com/art_expertyou.html, accessed March 26, 2007; Shery Mead and Mary Ellen Copeland. "What Recovery Means to Us," 2000, Plenum Publishers, New York, www.mentalhealthrecovery.com/art_recoverymeans_php, accessed March 26, 2007.
33. Clinical Guide 23, "Depression: Management of Depression in Primary and Secondary Care," National Institute for Clinical Excellence, National Health Service (UK), December 2004.

CHAPTER SEVEN: THE SEA SNAIL SYNDROME

1. William H. Calvin, *The Throwing Madonna: Essays on the Brain* (New York: McGraw-Hill, 1983).
2. Eric R. Kandel, *In Search of Memory: The Emergence of a New Science of Mind* (New York: W. W. Norton, 2006), p. 55.
3. Interview with Eric Kandel, "The Future of Memory," *Molecular Interventions*, vol. 5, 2005, pp. 65–69.
4. Steve Mirsky, "The Future of Psychiatry: Eric Kandel Says It Lies With Biology," *Howard Hughes Medical Institute Bulletin*, vol. 3, no. 2 (September 2000) 6–8.
5. Kandel, p. 55.
6. Ibid., p. 145.
7. Eric. R. Kandel, autobiography, www.nobelprize.org, accessed August 1, 2007.
8. Kandel interview: "The Future of Memory," *Molecular Interventions.*
9. Kandel, *In Search of Memory*, p. 194.
10. Nancy Touchette, "How Sea Slugs Make Memories," *Genome News Network*, January 9, 2004.
11. Mirsky, "The Future of Psychiatry."
12. Kandel, *In Search of Memory*, p. 171.
13. Norman Doidge, "A Victory for Hope: Nobel Prize Winner Eric Kandel Has Revolutionized Our Understanding of the Brain," *National Post* (Canada), reprinted by The Gairdner Foundation, oct 25 2000, www.gairdner.org/news12.html, accessed July 1, 2004.
14. Eric R. Kandel, "A New Intellectual Framework for Psychiatry," Special Article, *American Journal of Psychiatry*, 155: 457–69, April 1998.
15. Kandel, "The Future of Memory."
16. Norman Doidge, *The Brain That Changes Itself: Stories of Personal Triumph from the Frontiers of Brain Science* (New York: Viking, 2007), p. 220.
17. BBC News, "Taxi Drivers' Brains 'Grow' on the Job," March 14, 2000.
18. H. Van Praag, G. Kempermann, and F. H. Gage, "Neural Consequences of Environmental Enrichment," *Nature Reviews: Neuroscience*, vol. 1, December 2000, 191–98); D. Y. Liggan and J. Kay, "Some Neurobiologi-

cal Aspects of Psychotherapy: A Review," *Journal of Psychotherapy Practice and Research*, vol. 8, April 1999, 103–14.

19. Leon Eisenberg, "Experience, Brain, and Behavior: The Importance of a Head Start," *Pediatrics*, vol. 103, no. 5 (May 1999), 1031–35.
20. L.R. Baxter, J.M. Schwartz, K.S. Bergman, et al., "Caudate Glucose Metabolic Rate Changes with Both Drug & Behavior Therapy for Obsessive-Compulsive Disorder," *Archives of General Psychiatry*, vol. 49, no. 9, 1992, 681–89. A. L. Brody, S. Saxena, P. Stoessel, L. A. Gillies, L. A. Fairbanks, S. Alborzian, M. E. Phelps, et al., "Regional Brain Metabolic Changes in Patients with Major Depression Treated with Either Paroxetine or Interpersonal Therapy: Preliminary Findings," *Archives of General Psychiatry*, vol. 58, no. 7, July 2001, 631–40.
21. David Dobbs, "Profile: Helen Mayberg: Turning Off Depression," *Scientific American Mind*, August/September 2006.
22. Eric Kandel, "A New Intellectual Framework for Psychiatry," *American Journal of Psychiatry* 155, no. 44, 1998, 457–69.
23. Liggan and Kay, "Some Neurobiological Aspects of Psychotherapy; A Review," April 1999.
24. A. Etkin, C. Pittenger, H. J. Polan, and E. R. Kandel, "Toward a Neurobiology of Psychotherapy: Basic Science and Clinical Applications," *The Journal of Neuropsychiatry and Clinical Neurosciences*, vol. 17, May 2005, 145–58.
25. Steven Arnold, personal correspondence, August 20, 2007.
26. Glen O. Gabbard, "A Neurobiologically Informed Perspective on Psychotherapy," *British Journal of Psychiatry*, vol. 177, 2000, 117–22.
27. Leon Eisenberg, "Nature, Niche and Nurture: The Role of Social Experience in Transforming Genotype into Phenotype," *Academic Psychiatry*, vol. 22, December 1998, 213–22.
28. Ibid.
29. Ibid.
30. J. T. Cacioppo, G. G. Bernston, and R. Adolphs, eds., *Foundations in Social Neuroscience* (Cambridge, MA: MIT Press, 2002).
31. Goleman, *Social Intelligence*, p. 10.
32. Beth Azar, "At the Frontier of Science: Social Cognitive Neuroscience

Merges Three Distinct Disciplines in Hopes of Deciphering the Process Behind Social Behavior," *Monitor on Psychology*, vol. 33, no. 1, January 2002, www.apa.org/monitor/jan02/frontier.html, accessed January 10, 2007.

33. A. Raine, K. Mellingen, J. Liu, et al., "Effects of Environmental Enrichment at Ages 3–5 Years on Schizotypal Personality and Antisocial Behavior at Ages 17 and 23 Years," *American Journal of Psychiatry*, vol. 160, 2003, 1627–35.
34. Aditi Eleswarapu, "In Rat Race, Running in Groups More Effective," *The Daily Princetonian*, March 17, 2006, www.dailyprincetonian.com/archives/2006/03/17/news/14907.shtml, accessed October 12, 2007.
35. E. Susser, E. Valencia, S. Conover, A. Felix, W. Y. Tsai, and R. J. Wyatt, "Preventing Recurrent Homelessness Among Mentally Ill Men: A Critical Time Intervention After Discharge from a Shelter," *American Journal of Public Health*, vol. 87, issue 2, 1997, 256–62.
36. D. Herman, L. Opler, A. Felix, E. Valenica, R. J. Wyatt, and E. Susser, "A Critical Time Intervention with Mentally Ill Homeless Men: Impact on Psychiatric Symptoms," *Journal of Nervous and Mental Disease*, vol. 188, no. 3, March 2000, 135–40.

POSTSCRIPT: EMOTIONAL RESCUE

1. Jay Tolson, *Pilgrim in the Ruins: A Life of Walker Percy* (New York: Simon & Schuster, 1992), p. 51.
2. Carl Olson, "Traveling with Walker Percy," *Saint Austin Review*, 2003, www.ignatiusinsight.com/Features/ceolson_walkerpercy_nov04.asp., November 2004, accessed August 20, 2007.
3. Ralph C. Wood (Baylor University), An Introduction to Walker Percy. www3.baylor.edu/~Ralph_Wood/percy/IntroductionPercy.pdf, accessed February 12, 2007.
4. Olson, "Traveling with Walker Percy," 2003.
5. Percy, *Lost in the Cosmos: The Last Self-Help Book* (New York: Picador, 2000), p. 76.
6. Martin Seligman Forum on Depression, interview by Julie McGrossin.

7. Kathryn Schulz, "Did Antidepressants Depress Japan?" *The New York Times*, August 22, 2004.
8. Ibid.
9. Ibid.
10. James Joyce, *A Portrait of the Artist As a Young Man*, (New York: B. W. Huebsch, 1916), p. 168.
11. Scott Raab, "Steve Earle, Folk Hero," *Esquire*, June 1, 2000.
12. Marsha Barber, "Their Own Damn Selves: Museum Spotlights Hometown Work," *Mountain Xpress* (Asheville, NC), vol. 7, no. 23, January 17, 2001.
13. Rainer Maria Rilke, *Ahead of All Parting: The Selected Poetry and Prose of Rainer Maria Rilke*, ed. and trans. Stephen Mitchell (New York: Modern Library, 1995).
14. Jim Rosack, "Companies Desperately Seek Antidepressant Breakthrough," *Psychiatric News*, vol. 41, no. 11, June 2, 2006, 22.
15. Glen Gabbard, personal correspondence, February 1, 2007.
16. T. M. Luhrmann, *Of Two Minds: An Anthropologist Looks at American Psychiatry*, p. 212.

Index

Abilify, 87
Abramawitz, Jonathan, 153
acceptance, 162, 184–85
achievement, 220–21
addictions 26, 54–55
  in homeless population, xi, 169–70, 204, 206–7, 210
Adler, Alfred, 141
advertising, direct-to-consumer, 33, 45–49, 101, 102, 135
Agee, James, 217
Agency for Health Care Policy and Research, U.S., 52
akathisia, 88–89
Albert Lasker Clinical Medical Research Award, 160
Alcoholics Anonymous (AA), 169, 172, 180
alcoholism, xi, 25, 173
Allegra, 49
Alline, Henry, 109
all-or-nothing thinking, 142
Alzheimer's disease, 23
Ambien, 41, 46
ambivalence, 173, 174, 177, 178
American Medical Association, 44
American Psychiatric Association, 28, 47, 52, 69, 71, 105, 119–20
Ames, Rebecca, 47
amyotrophic lateral sclerosis, 40
Anafranil, 8
Angell, Marcia, 32
anger, 123–24, 217
Annie Hall, 216–17
Anthony, William, 184
antidepressant discontinuation syndrome, 55–56
antidepressant drugs, xiv, 14, 20
  efficacy of, xviii–xix, 153, 190
  FDA database of, 52
  as lifestyle agents, 50, 105–6
  online availability of, 102–3
  overuse of, 5–6, 8–9, 100–107, 214–15
  suicidal thinking and, 102
  see also SSRIs; *specific drugs*

antipsychotic drugs, xii, xiii–xix, 8, 24, 84
side effects of, 77, 87–90
antisocial disorder, 202, 203
anxiety, 135, 157, 217
Aplysia californica, (sea snail), 191–96, 201
Archives of General Psychiatry, 123
Arfonad, 25
Arnold, Steven, 200
As Good as It Gets, 10, 11–12
Assertive Community Treatment (ACT) teams, 180
AstraZeneca, 13, 42, 44, 48
Asylum Psychiatry, 60–64, 65, 113
Ativan, 89
attention deficit hyperactivity disorder, 20, 28, 40
automatic thoughts, 141, 143–44, 149, 150
Awakenings, 11, 208

Barker, Pat, 71*n*
Barracks shelter, 204–7
Bassman, Ronald, 183
battle fatigue, 71
Bayer, 44
Beautiful Mind, A, xiv, 10, 11
Beck, Aaron, 139–47, 160, 164–66
Beck, Judith, 140, 143, 146, 147, 148, 160
Beck Diet Solution, The (Beck), 160
Beck Institute for Cognitive Therapy and Research, 140, 146, 148
Begley, Sharon, 80
behavioral health, as term, 147–48
behavioral techniques, 144–45
Bellevue Hospital Center, 13
Bell Jar, The (Plath), 16
benzodiazepines, xi, 25, 53, 54, 55, 84
Better Than Well (Elliott), 24
Betty (patient), 89–90
Beyond the Pleasure Principle (Freud), 75
Binswanger, Ludwig, 78
bipolar disorder, xi, xiii, 14, 18, 20, 39, 40, 57, 84, 92, 105, 113, 117, 153, 187, 215–16
Blashfield, Roger K., 119
borderline personality disorders, xiv, 117, 158, 161–63, 199
Bowling Alone (Putnam), 126
brain function, 67–68, 78–82, 94–98
effect of social experience on, 191, 196
neuronal changes in, xvii–xviii, 191, 193–200, 210
brain imaging, xvii, 75, 78–82, 199, 209
Brand Institute, 49–50
Bristol-Myers Squibb, 10, 23
British Empire, 133
British Medical Journal, 42, 52, 114*n*, 122–23
Brooks, Bryan, 93
Buddhism, 161, 162–63, 164–66
Bush, George H. W., 32, 78
Bush, George W., 32, 82, 179
Bush (GWB) administration, 23, 31, 32, 36
Business Week, 130

Cacioppo, John, 201
Caplan, Arthur, 44
Captain Newman, MD, 74
Card, Andrew, 33

cardiovascular disease, 23, 184
Carli, Thomas, 38
Carlyle, Thomas, 131
catastrophizing, 142, 147
Cat's Cradle (Vonnegut), 23
Cattell, Dinah, 43
caudate nucleus, 198, 199
Celebrex, 45, 49
C. elegans (roundworm), 95
Celexa, 24, 52, 93
Center for Cognitive Neuroscience, 68
Center for Cognitive Therapy, 145
Center for Neurobiology and Behavior, 68
Center for Policy Alternatives, 37
Center for Science in the Public Interest, 36
Center for the Study of Brain, Mind and Behavior, 68
centering prayer, 162
Centers for Disease Control, 106, 111
central nervous system diseases, *see* mental illness, severe change, 168, 224
  Motivational Interviewing and, 173–79
  stages of, xvii, 169–73, 179, 186
Cheever, John, 126
children and adolescents, xvi, 43, 54, 90–92
chronic paranoid schizophrenia, 88
Cialis, 50
Clarinex, 49
Claritin, 45, 49
clients, *see* patients
clinical trials, 34–35, 40–41, 43–44, 66–67, 152
Clinton, Bill, xiv, 32
Clockwork Orange, A, 68
Clomicalm, 8
Clozaril, xii, 88
cocaine, xi, 65, 91
cocooning, 127
cognitive-behavioral therapy (CBT), xvi–xvii, 92, 135, 140–55, 189
  acceptance of, 159–61
  automatic thoughts and, 141, 143–44, 149, 150
  Buddhism and, 161, 162–63, 164–66
  core and intermediate beliefs in, 143–44, 149, 150
  criminal recidivism and, 154–55
  depression and, 141–42, 148–51, 152, 198
  efficacy of, 152–55, 166–67
  hard work of, 166–67
  suicidal behavior and, 146, 148–50, 153–54
  thinking errors codified in, 142–43
colleges and universities, drug company funding for, 44
college students, 16–17
Colombia, 19
Columbia University, 69
community integration, 182, 183
  see also social support
Community Mental Health Act (1963), 29, 65
Community Psychiatry, 60, 61, 64–65
compulsive shopping disorder, 124
Consumers Union, 33
Copeland, Mary Ellen, 187–88
core beliefs, 143–44, 149, 150

Corporate Psychiatry, 60, 61, 65, 155, 158
cortisol, 197
Cotton, Henry, 62
crack, xi, 27, 65, 204, 206, 210
Crawford, Lester M., 32
Crick, Francis, 83
criminal recidivism, 154–55
crisis counseling, 159
CT scans, 78
Curtis, John, 209–10
Cymbalta, 14

Dalai Lama, 161, 164–65
Dalmane, 25
Daniels, Mitch, 23
Darwin, Charles, 191
data mining, 37
Davidson, Larry, 183, 186
DBT (Dialectical Behavioral Therapy), 163–64
"Decade of the Brain, The," 78, 95
Defoe, Daniel, 62
Delano, Frank, 50
Delay, Jean, 68
dementia, 39
Deniker, Pierre, 76–77
Depakote, xiii, 85, 86, 87
depression, xiii, 14, 19, 106–7, 155
  monamine theory of, 97–98
  psychotherapeutic vs. pharmacological treatments of, 103–5, 151
  SSRIs and, 95–98
depression, major (clinical), xi, 20, 51, 84, 95, 105, 113, 150, 157, 215–16
  diagnosis of, 107–8, 110–12
depression, subsyndromal, 16–17, 100–107, 135, 215–18
  CBT and, 141–42, 148–51, 198
  Motivational Interviewing and, 178–79
  SSRIs and, xiii, 8, 28, 51–53, 198
  treatment guidelines for, 52–53, 189–90
DeRubeis, Robert, 153
detailers, 37, 38
Detorre, James L., 49–50
Deutsch, Albert, 62
diabetes, xi, xix, 39, 184
Diagnostic and Statistical Manual of Mental Disorders, see DSM
Dialectical Behavioral Therapy (DBT), 163–64
Dickinson, Emily, 109–10
DiClemente, Carlo, 170, 173, 174
diet, 155–56, 202–4
DiFebo, Val, 48
direct-to-consumer (DTC) advertising, 33, 45–49, 101, 102, 135
discounting positives, 142
"disease," 118–19
"disorder," 118–20
doctor-patient relationship, 168–69
doctors:
  drug company gifts and marketing to, 37–38, 44
  primary care, 112, 178
dogs, SSRIs prescribed for, 7, 8
Doidge, Norman, 195
dopamine, 90, 96
drug abuse, 24–25
drug safety, FDA and, 33–36
drug sales representatives, 37, 38
DSM *(Diagnostic and Statistical*

Manual of Mental Disorders), 28, 121–22
DSM-I, 113, 117
DSM-II, 113, 117, 118
DSM-III, 113, 117–18
DSM-IV, 113, 119–20
DSM-V, 113, 119
Duino Elegies, The (Rilke), 221
Duman, Ronald, 97

Eagleton, Thomas, 18
Earle, Steve, 220–21
education, 202–4
Effexor, 14, 24, 50, 52, 55–56
ego, 193, 195
Eisenberg, Leon, 70, 201
electroconvulsive therapy, 109
Eli Lilly, 7, 23, 24, 26, 34, 38, 39, 40–41, 44
Elliott, Carl, 24, 114
Ellis, Albert, 146
emotional contrasts, 219–22
emotional entitlement, 129–32
emotional reasoning, 142
empathy, of therapists, 168, 173–74, 175
English Men of Science (Galton), 200–201
enrichment programs, 202–4
Epictetus, 141
epilepsy, 40
Erikson, Erik, 139, 185
Evans, Richard, 45
exercise, 155, 156

FDA (U.S. Food and Drug Administration), 32–36, 45, 52
clinical trial standards of, 34–35, 41
drug regulation by, 7, 8, 31–36, 39, 40, 46, 51, 77, 105
SSRI suicide risk warning of, xvi
Fenton, Lisa, 147–51
Fincham, Jack, 106
fish oil, in brain health, 155–56, 167, 257
flaming, 15
Flügel, Fritz, 78
fluoxetine, *see* Prozac
flu vaccines, 23
fMRI (Functional Magnetic Resonance Imaging), 79–80, 196, 200
Food and Drug Administration, U.S., *see* FDA
Frances, Allen, 118
Franklin, David P., 40
Freedman, Joshua, 82
Freedman, Robert, xix
Freedom of Information Act, 52
Freeman, Walter, 63–64
Freud, Sigmund, 70, 72, 75, 113, 117, 146, 193
Fugh-Berman, Adriane, 42

GABA (gamma-aminobutyric acid), 96, 98
Gabbard, Glen, 156, 222
Galton, Francis, 200–201
Gazzaniga, Michael, 75, 80
generalized anxiety disorder, 28, 46–47, 59
General Motors, 13
genes, 195–96, 201
George, Kate, 222
Georgia, 179–80
Gesch, Bernard, 155
Girl, Interrupted, 10, 12

GlaxoSmithKline, 9, 34, 44, 46–47, 54, 119, 218
glial cells, 95, 197
glutamate, 98
Good Life and Its Discontents, The (Samuelson), 129–30
Good Will Hunting, 10, 12
Gourevitch, Marc, 177–78
Greenson, Ralph, 74
group therapy, 73
Grundfest, Harry, 193
Gulf War, 197

habituation, 193–94
Haldol (haloperidol), xii, 26, 49, 88, 89, 206–7, 210
happiness, pressure for, 129–32
Harding, Courtenay, 181–82, 184, 186, 187
Hartford Retreat, 60
Harvard University, 17, 123–24
Health and Human Services Department, U.S., 31
health care costs, 30
Healy, David, 43, 50–51, 54–55, 58, 112
hepatitis, xi, 184
heroin, xi, 27
hippocampus, 97, 197
hippocratic oath, 44
HIV/AIDS, xi, 27, 184
Hoffman-La Roche Inc., 25
Holmes, Oliver Wendell, 62
homeless population, 219
  addictions in, xi, 204, 206–7, 210
  mental illness in, xi–xiii, xviii–xix, 65, 169–70, 205–10
  in shelters, 65, 205–7
Horney, Karen, 146
hospitalization, xix, 24
Hughes, Howard, 69
Human Genome Project, 66
Hyman, Steven, 81
hyperactivity, 91
hypnotics, 54
hypomania, xiii, 18
Hypomanic Edge, The, 17
hypothalamus, 90

id, 193, 195
identity problem, 120
illness, 118–19
  as part of human condition, 224–25
IMS Health, 37, 222
India, 34–35, 87
individualism, 131, 133
Insel, Thomas, 34, 154
insomnia, 14, 28, 41, 54
  CBT and, 152
  SSRIs and, 54
Integrated Behavioral Health, 160
intermediate beliefs, 143–44, 150
inward turning, 132–35
Iraq War, 14, 71
Ireland, 87
isolation, 126–28
"issues," as euphemism, 18
Italians, 19

Jacobson, Michael F., 36
Japan, 218
Jefferson, Thomas, 131
Johnson, Lyndon, 29
Johnson & Johnson, 13, 24, 40–41
José (counselor), 205–7, 210
journal articles, ghost-written, 41–43

Journal of Happiness Studies, 132
Journal of Neuroscience, 69
Journal of Pain, 154
Journal of the American Medical Association, 42, 102, 152
Joyce, James, 219–20
"Julie," 100–105, 111–12, 120–21, 124–26, 134, 213, 214, 222
Jung, Carl, 70, 146
Justice Department, U.S., 39–40

Kaiser Permanente, 104
Kandel, Eric, 83, 95, 192–99
Katrina, Hurricane, 14, 159
Kawai, Hayao, 218
Kennedy, John F., 29, 65, 75
Kessler, David, 32
Kessler, Ronald, 124
Khan, Arif, 52
Klonopin, 25, 53
Kraepelin, Emil, 181, 182
Kramer, Peter, xv, 20, 53, 58

Laborit, Henri, 76
Lamictal, 92
Lancet, 42
Layard, Lord, 160–61
learning, biology of, 193–200
Leary, Timothy, 104
Lehman, Heinz, 68, 76
Lennon, John, 28, 85
Lexapro, 8, 14, 24
Licinio, Julio, 53
lifestyle agents, xv, 50, 105–6
Light, Paul, 32–33
lightning-bolt syndrome, 55
Lincoln's Melancholy, 17
Linehan, Marsha, 161, 162–64
Lipitor, xv, 49, 87
Listening to Prozac (Kramer), xv, 20, 53
lithium, xii, xiii, 26, 85, 86, 88
lobotomies, 63–64
London taxi drivers, neuronal change in, 197
Lost in the Cosmos (Percy), 212, 216
Lou Gehrig's disease, 40
LSD, 27, 28
Luhrmann, T. M., 8, 75, 224
Lunesta, 41, 46

MacArthur Foundation, 116
McCall, Timothy B., 104
MacDonald, Angus, III, 200
McGill University, 68, 76
McHugh, Paul, 108
McKenzie, D. Banks, 179
McKinnell, Henry, 59
McMahon, Darrin M., 131
Madison County, Iowa, 4–5
Maguire, Eleanor, 197
managed care, xix, 65, 103–5, 157
Manhattan State Psychiatric Hospital, 60, 77
manic states, 57
Mann, John J., 108
Mansfield, Harvey, 28
MAOI antidepressants, xiv, 84
Marcus Aurelius, 141
marijuana, 27, 28
marketing, by drug companies, 6–8, 23–24, 36–40, 166, 218
  brand names and, 49–50
  direct-to-consumer advertising in, 33, 45–49, 101, 102, 135
Marshall, George, 73
Marshall, Mary Faith, 32
Martha (patient), 148–51

Masters, Scott, 41, 51
Mauritius, 202–3
media, xviii, 14–15
Medicaid, 130, 180
Medicare, 39, 130
Mencken, H. L., 108
Menninger, Karl, 74, 113
Menninger, William, 72–73, 113
Menninger Foundation, 74
Mental Health Act (1946), 73
mental hygiene movement, 71
mental illness, xii–xvii, 18–19
  diet and, 155–56, 202–4
  exercise and, 155, 156, 202–4
  as marketing opportunities, 23–24, 47
  media portrayal of, 14–15
  in movies, 10–12
  mystery and complexity of, 222–25
  in popular culture, xiv–xv, 9–21
  self-reported incidence of, 19
mental illness, severe, xi, xiii, xiv–xv, xviii–xix, 10, 13, 16, 20–21, 84–90, 105, 215–16
  biological bases of, 67–68
  chronic nature of, 23–24, 184
  environmental explanations of, 68
  genetic bases of, 66, 68
  in homeless population, xi–xiii, 65, 169–70, 205–10
  insufficient care for, 115–16
  recovery from, 181, 183–84
  research on, 115–16
  suicide and, 116–17
  see also specific diseases
Merck, 22, 23
Mexicans, 19
Meyer, Adolf, 62
Meyer, Jeffrey, 98
migraine, 40
military, U.S., psychiatry and, 72–73, 158, 179
Miller, William R., 173–78
Millie (patient), 84–87, 90
mindfulness, 161, 163
mind reading, 143
mirror neurons, 15
misery, 125–35
mixed states, 57
Moniz, Egas, 63
monoamine theory, 97–98
mood stabilizers, xii, 84
moon exploration, 134
"Mother's Little Helper," 25
motivation, 174–75, 178, 224
motivational deficiency disorder (spoof), 122–23
Motivational Interviewing (MI), xvii, 169, 173–79, 186
Mount Sinai Hospital, 85–86
movies, mental illness portrayed in, 10–12
MRI (Magnetic Resonance Imaging) scans, 78, 81–82
mutation, 195

Narcotics Anonymous (NA), 169, 172, 180
national catastrophes, mental component of, 13–14, 47
National Health Service, British, 160–61
National Institute for Health and Clinical Excellence, British, 189–90
National Institute of Mental Health (NIMH), 34, 69, 73, 115, 166

National Institutes of Health, 39, 201–2
Naturalis Historia (Pliny), 191
nature vs. nurture, 200–201
nefazodone, 43
Netherlands, 55
neurobiology, 14–16
neuroleptic malignant syndrome, 89–90
neurons, neuronal change, xvii–xviii, 15, 94–95, 191, 193–200, 210, 222
Neurontin, 40, 87
neuroplasticity, 195, 197, 198, 200
neuropsychiatry, *see* psychiatry, biological
neuroscience, 68–70, 82, 193, 222
  lived experience vs., 222–23
  social, 201–4, 210
neuroses, *see* psychological distress
neurotransmitters, 67, 96–97
New England Journal of Medicine, 17, 42, 43, 62
"New Intellectual Framework for Psychiatry, A" (Kandel), 195, 198–99
New York, N.Y., xi, xviii
New York Times, 15–16, 19, 30, 41, 48, 62, 80, 81, 104
Nexium, 48–49
Nietzche, Friedrich, 223
Nigerians, 19
NIMH (National Institute of Mental Health), 34, 69, 73, 115, 166
norepinephrine, 96
not otherwise specified (NOS), 121–22
Novartis, 13, 34
obsessive-compulsive disorder (OCD), 28, 105, 198
  CBT and, 152, 198
occupational disorder, 120
off-label drug uses, 39–40, 56
Okun, Arthur, 125
omega-3 fatty acids, 155, 203
online disinhibition effect, 15
Opler, Lewis, 155
orbitofrontal cortex, 15
outsourcing, 87
  of clinical trials, 34–35
overgeneralization, 143

Pace, Alison, 48
pain, 154
  as part of human condition, 224–25
  pleasure linked to, 219–22
parent-child relationships, 121
Parkinson's disease, 23
patent life, 30–31, 41
patients:
  doctor's relationship with, 168–69
  responsibility of, 175, 177, 186–89
  strengths and resources of, 185, 188–89
Paxil, xii, xiii, xv, 6, 52, 93
  marketing of, 45, 46–47, 50, 53, 119, 218
  withdrawal problems with, 54–56
pediatric psychopharmacology, 43
peer engagement, 179–80
Pendergast, Mary, 33
Pennsylvania, University of, Center for Cognitive Therapy at, 145, 164–66
Percy, Walker, 93–94, 133, 211–14, 220

Percy, William, 211
Percy family, 211–12
performance pressure, SSRIs and, 27–28
Perrin, Jean, 76
personality disorders, xi
personalization, 143
PET (Positron Emission Tomography) scans, 78–79
Pfizer, 10, 22, 23, 34, 39, 44, 59, 87
pharmacology industry, 87
  clinical trials funded by, 40, 43–44
  FDA regulation of, 7, 8, 31–36, 39, 40, 46, 51, 77, 105
  marketing by, *see* marketing, by drug companies
  profits in, xv–xvi, 22–24, 30–31, 44, 59
  public perception of, 44–45, 59
  research budgets of, 36, 38
Philadelphia Psychoanalytic Institute, 139
phobias, 28, 145, 152
Pinker, Steven, 79, 82
placebo effect, 83–84
Plath, Sylvia, 16, 63
pleasure, pain linked to, 219–22
Pliny the Elder, 191
Pogues, the, 212
Pomerantz, Jay, 52, 53
popular culture, xviii
  mental illness in, xiv–xv, 9–21
Portrait of the Artist as a Young Man (Joyce), 219–20
posttraumatic stress disorder, 14, 71, 73, 199
prefrontal cortex, 63, 200, 209, 210
premature ejaculation, 28
prescriber reports, 37
prescription drug sales, in U.S. vs. worldwide, 20
Prescription Drug User Fee Act (PDUFA; 1992), 31–32
Prochaska, James, 170
Prolixin, 85, 86
Prozac (fluoxetine), xii, xiii, xv, 6, 38, 47, 51, 52, 56, 61, 92–93, 106, 149
  introduction of, 7–8, 24–25, 26, 46
  marketing of, 49–50
  in water supply, 92–93
Prozac Sisters, 10
psychedelic drugs, 27
psychiatric chic, 16
psychiatric drugs, 26–27
  children and, 90–92
  efficacy of, xviii–xix, 75
  increased use of, xv, 5–6, 90, 223–24
  as primary source of drug company profits, 23–24
  psychotherapy vs., 156–57, 167
  U.S. vs. worldwide use of, 20
  see also SSRIs; *specific drugs*
Psychiatric News, 47, 105
psychiatry, 65–66, 75, 87–88
  asylum era of, 60–64, 65, 113
  community era of, 60, 61, 64–65
  corporate era of, 60, 61, 65, 155, 158
  increased visibility of, 61, 73–75
  U.S. military and, 72–73, 158, 179
  see also mental illness
psychiatry, biological, xviii, 65–70, 75–84, 222–23
  enthusiasm for, 82–84, 94, 224
  see also neuroscience

psychoanalysis, 64, 70–75, 78, 142, 146, 157, 158, 159, 193
psychological distress, 112–16
see also specific disorders
Psychology of *The Sopranos* (Gabbard), 156
psychopharmacology, 68
psychotherapy:
cost effectiveness of, 157–58
efficacy of, 166–67, 198–200
hard work of, 166–67, 224
medications vs., 156–57, 167
neuronal change and, 198–200
schizophrenia and, 157
see also psychoanalysis; *specific therapies*
Puerto Rico, drug manufacturing outsourced to, 87
Pug Hill, 48
puritanism vs. excess, in American character, 20
Putnam, Robert, 126

Rabinow, Paul, 66
rats, learning in, 197
Reagan, Ronald, 5, 27, 29, 130
recovered memories, 158–59
recovery, recovery movement, 180–89
reentry, Percy's concept of, 212–15
reflective listening, 176–77
Regeneration (Barker), 71*n*
relapse, 171, 172
relational problem—not otherwise specified, 121
Remeron, 52
Report on Mental Health (U.S. Surgeon General), 105
research, on mental illness, 115–16
responsibility, of patient, 175, 177, 186–89
restless-leg syndrome, 40
retrospective diagnosis, 17–18
Rex (patient), 204–10
Rieff, Philip, 70
Rilke, Rainer Maria, 221
Risperdal, xii, 24, 41
Ritalin, 8, 91, 128
Rogers, Carl, 173
Rogers, Joseph A., 179
Rollnick, Steve, 174, 176, 177
Roosevelt, Theodore, 32, 36
Roper, Anthony, 223–24
Rose, Steven, 66
Rosenbaum, Jerrold, 159
Rosenblatt, Jack E., 41
Rozerem, 41
Rumsfeld, Donald, 23
RxComms, 42

Sacher, David, 83
Sacks, Oliver, 208
sadness, in Japanese culture, 218
Sakel, Manfred, 63
SAMHSA, 187
Samuelson, Robert J., 129–30
Sanacora, Gerard, 98
Schering-Plough, 44
schizophrenia, xi, xiii, xv, 13, 16, 20, 39, 70, 76–77, 78, 84, 88, 105, 111, 113, 146, 169, 200, 215–16
clinical trials of drugs for, 40–41, 67
psychotherapy and, 157
recovery from, 181, 183, 186–87
suicide and, 116–17
symptoms of, 209
SCID (Structured Clinical Interview for DSM), 112, 125

Scientific American, 69, 77, 82
Searle, 23
Searle, John, 83
sedatives, 54
seizures, 40
selective serotonin reuptake inhibitors, *see* SSRIs
self-efficacy, 175, 177
Seligman, Martin, 106, 126, 217
sensitization, 193–94
separation anxiety, in dogs, 7, 8
September 11, 2001 terrorist attacks, 14, 47, 82, 159
Seroquel, 24
serotonin, 55, 58, 95, 96, 97–98, 199
serotonin reuptake enhancers, 96
serotonin syndrome, 56
Serzone, 52
Shakespeare, William, 197
Shame of the States, The (Deutsch), 62
shell shock, 70–71
Shelton, Richard, 55
should and *must* statements, 143
sibling relational problem, 121
Sinclair, Upton, 32
Skinner, B. F., 144, 146
Sleeping Father, The (Sharpe), 10
sleeping pills, 92
Smith, Patrick, 48
Smith Kline & French, 77
social anxiety disorder, 7, 28, 47
social programs, 29
Social Security, 29, 130
social service agencies, 64, 185–86
social support, 157, 174–75, 182–84
Society for Neuroscience, 69
Southern California, University of, 202–3
space program, 29
SPECT (Single Photon Emission Computed Tomography) scans, 78
Spitzer, Robert, 117–18
SSRIs (selective serotonin reuptake inhibitors), 28–29, 84
  addictiveness of, 54–55
  efficacy of, 50–53
  emotional entitlement and, 129
  marketing of, 6–8, 218
  mechanism of, 95–98
  numbing effect of, 6
  off-label uses of, 56, 105–6, 124
  overuse of, xiv–xvi, 8–9, 114, 124–25, 190, 198, 214–15, 223
  popular acceptance of, 27–30
  prenatal exposure to, 58
  profitability of, 30
  side effects of, 53–58
  and suicidal thinking, xvi, 43, 51
  withdrawal problems with, 54–57
  see also specific drugs
Stages of Change model, xvii, 169–73, 179, 186
Stanford University, 124
Steere, William C., 22
sterilization, of psychiatric patients, 62
Sternbach, Leo, 25
Stoic philosophers, 141
Stoll, Andrew, 155
Strauss, John, 186–87
Structured Clinical Interview for DSM (SCID), 112, 125
Styron, William, 107, 183
Substance Abuse and Mental Health Services Administration, 187

suicidal behavior, 102, 162, 211–12
CBT and, 146, 148–50, 153–54
SSRIs and, xvi, 43, 51
Sullivan, Harry Stack, 71, 179
Summers, Larry, 17
superego, 193, 195
Susann, Jacqueline, 25–26
Sussman, Norman, 54

Takahashi, Tohru, 218
Talbot, John, 63
tardive dyskinesia, 88
Taxi Driver, 11, 12
taxi drivers, neuronal change in, 197
television, 12–13, 128
Thanatos Syndrome, The, 93–94
therapies, nonpharmaceutic, xvi–xvii
declining use of, 29
see also specific therapies
Thorazine, xii, 26, 61, 64, 68, 75–78, 88
Three Faces of Eve, The, 11, 74
3M Company, 69
tianeptine, 96
Tillotson, Kenneth, 63
Time, 13, 14, 17, 72, 92, 130
Tintin, 210
tobacco industry, 32
Tom (patient), 88
Topeka Psychoanalytic Society, 72
transcriptional function, of genes, 196
trauma, 197
trazodone, 41
Treating Addictive Behaviors (Miller et al.), 173
tricyclics, 53
Trilling, Lionel, 70
Trombetta, Bill, 49–50
Turner, Frederick Jackson, 132–34
twelve-step programs, 169, 172, 180

Ukraine, 19
Union of Concerned Scientists, 35
US News & World Report, 130

Vaillant, George, 185
Valenstein, Elliot, 96–97
Valium, 25–27, 53, 61, 93, 106
addictiveness of, 26
Valley of the Dolls (Susann), 26
Vaughan, Bill, 33
Vermont State Hospital, 181–82
Viagra, xv, 45, 46, 49, 50, 87
Vietnam War, 65, 71, 197
Vioxx, 23, 33
Virtual Prozac, 10
Vonnegut, Kurt, 23
Voyage of the Beagle, The (Darwin), 191

Wall Street Journal, 80
Walsh, Timothy, 84
Warfarin, 42
Warner-Lambert, 39–40
Waxman, Henry A., 36
Wellbutrin, 9, 14, 50, 52, 87
Wellmark Blue Cross and Blue Shield, 5
Wellness Recovery Action Plan, The (Copeland), 188–89
Westen, Drew, 159
whistleblower suits, 40
Wiesel, Torsten, 95
Wiley, Harvey, 36
Williamson, T. Lynn, 38
Winterset, Iowa, 3–6, 8, 98, 224
withdrawal problems, from SSRIs, 54–57

Wolfe, Tom, 68
Wolpe, Paul Root, 81
Wonderland, 13
Wong, David, 7–8
Woodcock, Janet, 31
"Woody Allen syndrome," 70
work, in psychotherapy, 166–67, 224
World Congress of Biological Psychiatry, 37–38
World Health Organization, 19, 54, 115, 123, 180, 181
World Trade Center, 47
World War I, 70–71
World War II, 71–73, 179
Wyeth, 24
Wyeth-Ayerst, 44

Xanax, 23

Yale-New Haven Hospital, 57
yawning-excitement syndrome, 54
Young, John, 76

Zen Buddhism, 162–63
Zoloft, xii, xiii, xv, 6, 7–8, 9, 14, 24, 43, 46, 51, 52, 87, 156
  marketing of, 45, 47–48, 49–50, 101, 106
  in water supply, 93
Zyprexa, xii, 9, 24, 38, 39, 41